GU00728921

ABBREV

AIDS	
ACMP	
BIS	British Infection Society
BNF	British National Formulary
CDC	Centers for Disease Control and Prevention
DEET	N,N diethyl-*m*-toluamide (an insect repellent)
EDTA	Ethylene diamine tetraacetic acid
FAQ	Frequently Asked Question
GP	General Practitioner
G6PD	Glucose 6-phosphate dehydrogenase (a metabolic enzyme)
HIV	Human Immunodeficiency Virus
HPA	Health Protection Agency
HTD	Hospital for Tropical Diseases
INR	International Normalized Ratio
IPS	International Passenger Survey
IPT	Intermittent Preventive Therapy
LSHTM	London School of Hygiene and Tropical Medicine
LSTM	Liverpool School of Tropical Medicine
NaTHNaC	National Travel Health Network and Centre
NNRTI	Non-Nucleoside Reverse Transcriptase Inhibitor
MHRA	Medicines and Healthcare products Regulatory Agency
MRL	Malaria Reference Laboratory
PI	Protease Inhibitor
PCR	Polymerase Chain Reaction
POM	Prescription Only Medicine
RDT	Rapid Diagnostic Test
RSTM&H	Royal Society of Tropical Medicine and Hygiene
SP	Sulfadoxine/pyrimethamine
SPC	Summary of Product Characteristics or 'data sheet'
UK	United Kingdom
VFR	Visiting Friends and Relatives
WHO	World Health Organization

Contents

Foreword   7

Chapter 1: General Issues   9
1.1   How to give the advice   11
1.2   Medical history of the traveller   11
1.3   Template for risk assessment and summary of advice given   12

Chapter 2: Awareness of Risk   17
2.1   What is malaria?   19
2.2   Life cycle   20
2.3   The malarial illness   21
2.4   Where is malaria found?   22
2.5   Level of risk of exposure to malaria and what affects it   22
2.6   Distribution of drug resistant malaria   23

Chapter 3: Bite Prevention   25
3.1   When do female Anopheles mosquitoes bite?   27
3.2   Measures to prevent mosquito bites   27
       3.2.1   Repellents   27
       3.2.2   Insecticides   28
       3.2.3   Nets   28
       3.2.4   Clothing   29
       3.2.5   Room protection   29
       3.2.6   Fallacies   29

Chapter 4: Chemoprophylaxis   31
4.1   Principles   33
4.2   The drugs   34
       4.2.1   Chloroquine   34
       4.2.2   Proguanil   35
       4.2.3   Chloroquine plus proguanil   36
       4.2.4   Mefloquine   36
       4.2.5   Doxycycline   37
       4.2.6   Atovaquone plus proguanil   38

Contents

4.3	Dosage tables	39
4.4	Country tables	42
4.5	Popular destinations	53
4.6	Emergency Standby Treatment	54

Chapter 5: Diagnosis — 59

5.1	Blood tests and how to request them	61
5.2	Rapid Diagnostic Tests (RDTs)	61
5.3	Blood film negative malaria	62
5.4	Resources for treatment advice	62
5.5	Notification	62

Chapter 6: Special Groups (Medical Conditions) — 63

6.1	Smoking cessation	65
6.2	Pregnancy	65
6.3	Breastfeeding	66
6.4	Anticoagulants	66
6.5	Epilepsy	67
6.6	Glucose 6-phosphate dehydrogenase deficiency	67
6.7	Sickle Cell disease	68
6.8	Immunocompromised Travellers	68
	6.8.1 Risks for transplant patients	68
	6.8.2 Risks for HIV/AIDS patients	68
6.9	Liver disease	69
6.10	Renal impairment	69
6.11	Splenectomy	70
6.12	Acute porphyrias	70

Chapter 7: Special Categories — 71

7.1	Children	73
7.2	Elderly travellers	74
7.3	Multi-trip travel	74

Contents

7.4	*Cruises*	74
7.5	*Oil rigs*	75
7.6	*Visits to national parks*	75
7.7	*Stopovers*	75
7.8	*Last minute travellers*	75
7.9	*Visiting friends and relatives*	76
7.10	*Students and children at boarding school*	77
7.11	*The long-term traveller*	77
	7.11.1 Risk assessment	77
	7.11.2 Chemoprophylaxis for long-term travellers	78
	7.11.3 Specific considerations for women	80
	7.11.4 Specific considerations for infants and older children	80
7.12	*Long term visitors to the UK returning to live in malarious parts of the world*	80
	7.12.1 Preventive measures appropriate to an endemic setting	82
	7.12.2 Prophylaxis	82
Chapter 8: Frequently Asked Questions		83
8.1	*What malaria prevention should be advised for travellers going on cruises?*	85
8.2	*What alternative antimalarial drugs can be used for India (and Sri Lanka) if chloroquine and proguanil are unsuitable for a traveller?*	85
8.3	*Which antimalarial can I give to a traveller with a history of psoriasis?*	86
8.4	*Which antimalarial can I give a traveller who is taking warfarin?*	86
8.5	*How long is it safe to continue a course of antimalarial tablets?*	87
8.6	*Which antimalarial drugs are suitable for women during pregnancy?*	88

Contents

8.7   Which antimalarial drugs can be taken by breastfeeding
        women?   89

8.8   Which malaria drugs can be given to babies and
        young children?   89

8.9   What is the easiest way to calculate the correct dose of
        chloroquine for babies and young children?   90

8.10   Many travellers I see intend to travel through several
        areas where different anti-malarials are recommended
        as they progress through their journey. How do we advise
        these travellers?   90

8.11   Which antimalarial drugs can I advise for a traveller
        who has epilepsy?   91

8.12   What do I advise for the traveller with Glucose 6-phosphate
        dehydrogenase deficiency?   91

8.13   What do I advise people working on oil rigs?   92

8.14   What do I advise for the traveller on a stopover?   92

Chapter 9: Information Resources   93

9.1   Expert centres   95
        9.1.1 Prophylaxis advice   95
        9.1.2 Diagnostic advice   95
        9.1.3 Treatment advice   95

9.2   Useful websites   95

9.3   Information leaflets   96

9.4   Reference list   97

Photograph courtesy of Jim Gathany/CDC

Foreword

Each year between 1500 and 2000 people are diagnosed with malaria on their return to the UK. Anyone visiting a malarious area can become infected no matter what age or sex or ethnic background. Malaria can kill very quickly if not diagnosed in time. In 2005 there were 11 deaths from malaria in the UK.

However these deaths and illness are avoidable. We know that most people requiring medical attention for malaria in the UK have not taken the correct precautions needed for their visit. The Health Protection Agency is committed to ensuring a continuing reduction in the risk of malaria to UK travellers by raising awareness of malaria before people travel and helping to guide healthcare professionals in giving the best advice available.

These guidelines from the Agency's Advisory Committee on Malaria Prevention in UK travellers update the 2003 advice. Both the web and book format have been designed with the busy health care advisor in mind so that they are easy to use and give clear simple guidance.

The general public may also find them useful to read before they visit their GP's surgery or a travel clinic for specific advice tailored to their needs; whether they are taking the children to visit family in Africa or India for a month, backpacking for 6 months round South America, taking a fortnight's package holiday to Africa or working for a week in the Middle East.

PROFESSOR PAT TROOP CBE

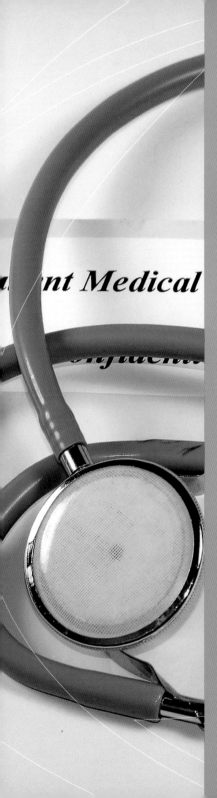

1 - General Issues

1.1
How to give the advice. 11

1.2
Medical history of the traveller. 11

1.3
Template for risk assessment
and summary of advice given. 12

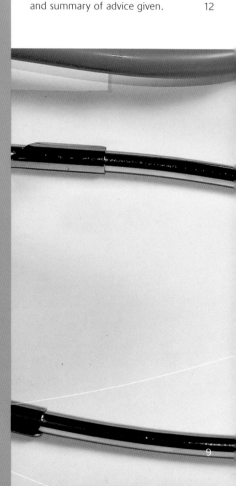

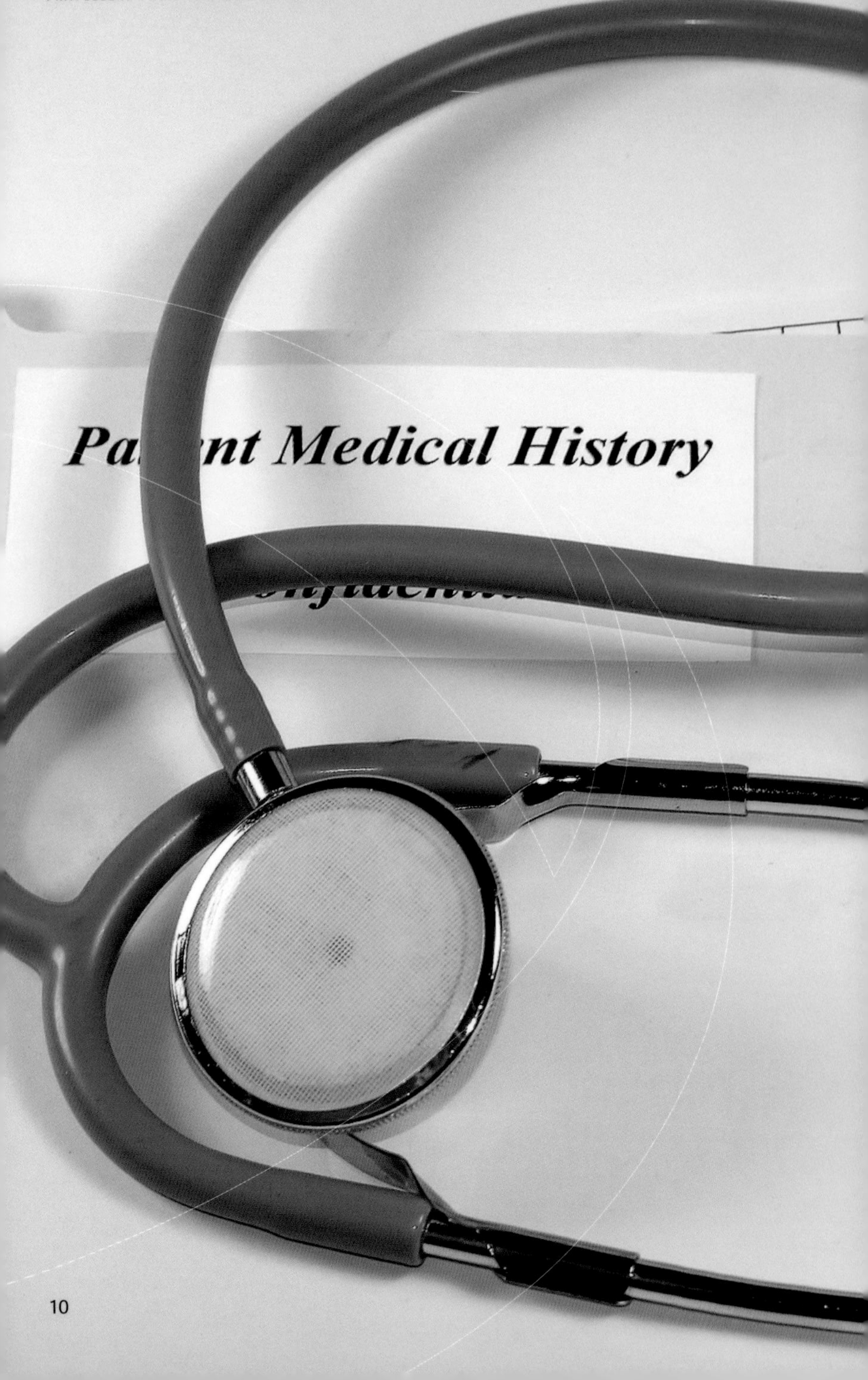
Pa nt Medical History

1. General Issues

The ACMP prophylaxis guidelines are intended for UK-based visitors to malaria endemic areas and may not be appropriate for use by those residing in endemic areas.

Whilst these guidelines deal with malaria, malaria prevention is only one aspect of pre-travel advice. An overall risk assessment-based package of travel health advice should be provided.

In these guidelines, which have been specifically developed for travellers from the UK, there are a small number of instances where the advice given differs from that in guidelines from other countries or the World Health Organization. This is because travellers from the UK do not usually visit all possible localities of malaria-endemic countries and may not visit the same localities as travellers from other countries. Many travellers from the UK who enter malaria-endemic countries are visiting friends and relatives in localities from which people tend to migrate to the UK. They do not therefore suffer exactly the same patterns of malaria exposure as permanent residents or visitors from other cultures.

1.1 How to give the advice

Emphasise to the traveller the ABCD of malaria prevention:
  Awareness of risk
  Bite prevention
  Chemoprophylaxis
  prompt **D**iagnosis and treatment

- Emphasise that whilst no regimen is 100% effective, the **combination** of preventive measures advised will give significant protection against malaria.

- Make use of visual aids, especially malaria distribution maps and show examples of the preventive measures advised, such as aids to bite prevention.

- Discuss the choices of chemoprophylaxis regimens and their individual advantages and disadvantages, including cost.

- Provide the traveller with written information on malaria and its prevention. The Department of Health has an information leaflet available in 11 different languages (see chapter 9).

1.2 Medical history of the traveller

It is essential that a full clinical history is obtained, to include current medication, significant health problems and any known drug allergies.

Safe and effective malaria prevention requires a sound knowledge of the medical history of the traveller. When their patients seek pre-travel advice in primary care, this information will be available from their own practice records but in the case of specialist travel clinics malaria prevention advice may be sought at the first attendance. The General Medical Council (2001)[1] states "If you provide treatment or advice for a patient, but are not the patient's general practitioner, you should tell the general practitioner the results of the investigations, the treatment provided and any other information necessary for the continuing care of the patient, unless the patient objects."

ACMP suggests that a hand-held record of the malaria prevention measures advised is given to the traveller so that they may pass it on to their GP.

1.3 Template for risk assessment and summary of advice given

This template is suggested for use in gathering information required for risk assessment when advising on malaria prevention. It may be downloaded for use from the Health Protection Agency website at www.hpa.org.uk or adapted for the particular circumstances of individual clinics.

Name

Age

Sex

Underlying condition:

Condition		Yes/No
Pregnancy	Actual	
	Planned while on trip	
Sickle cell	Disease	
	Carrier	
Thalassaemia	Disease	
	Carrier	
Epilepsy	Patient	
	First degree relative*	
Depression requiring medication		
Psychosis	Patient	
	First degree relative*	
Liver disease		
Renal failure		
Diabetes mellitus		
Cardiovascular	Ischaemic heart disease	
	Arrythmias	
	Other	
Immunocompromise		
Psoriasis		

* Note first degree relatives are included in risk assessment as a precaution since risk of epilepsy and major depression is higher in first degree relatives of those in whom these conditions have been diagnosed.

A condition in a first-degree relative may not contraindicate the use of an antimalarial, but may influence the choice of drug.

Allergies

Give details of allergies to drugs or other below

Medication

Current medication	Yes/No	Comments
Antiarrhythmics		
Anticonvulsants		
Anticoagulants		
Antiretrovirals		
Corticosteroids		
Oral contraceptives		
Bupropion (Zyban ®)		
Other		

Previous antimalarial chemoprophylactic agent taken	Describe any problems

Area to be visited
See country tables and maps

Destination	Length of stay	Risk of malaria	Urban/rural/ both	Prophylaxis advised from country table**

** If the recommended regimens differ between the countries to be visited, see note on multi-trips in chapter 7.

Purpose of visit and type of accommodation: tick those that apply

Visiting friends and relatives ☐	Safari ☐	Backpacking ☐
Business/work ☐	Study ☐	>6 months ☐	<6 months ☐
House ☐	Hotel ☐	Hostel ☐	Tent ☐
Oil Rig ☐	Cruise ship ☐	Urban ☐	Rural ☐
Other ☐ please give details below			

Advice given

Bite Prevention   Please tick measures advised

Repellent ☐   Clothing spray ☐   Bed net ☐

Coils / Electric vapourisers ☐   Insecticide sprays ☐

Chemoprophylaxis

Warning: do NOT rely on homoeopathic or 'natural' antimalarial prophylaxis

Antimalarial	Tick regimen advised	Dose	Duration	No. pills or volume of syrup
Chloroquine				
Proguanil				
Chloroquine/Proguanil				
Mefloquine				
Doxycycline				
Atovaquone/Progaunil				
Other (please specify)				
No chemoprophylaxis		Awareness of risk including bite prevention must still be recommended. Give advice to seek medical attention for any suspicious symptoms (up to about a year later)		

Standby Emergency Medication

For the vast majority of travellers standby emergency antimalarial medication is neither required nor recommended. Please undertake a risk assessment including information on the distance and time away from medical facilities which apply in each case.

Standby emergency medication advised?　Yes　/　No　　*Please circle*

If standby emergency medication is recommended, please tick the regimen advised

Atovaquone plus proguanil ☐　　　　Co-artemether ☐

Quinine plus doxycycline ☐　　　　Quinine plus clindamycin ☐

Standby emergency medication advice leaflet given　Yes　/　No　　*Please circle*

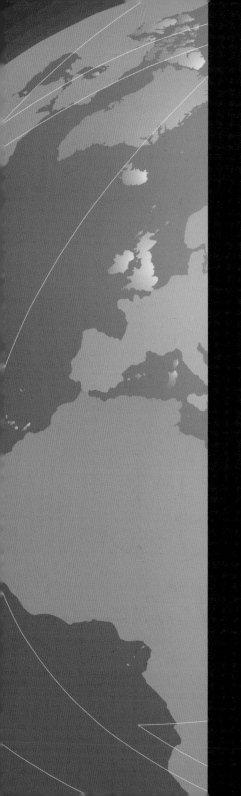

2 - Awareness of Risk

2.1
What is malaria?   19

2.2
Life cycle.   20

2.3
The malarial illness.   21

2.4
Where is malaria found?   22

2.5
Level of risk of exposure to
malaria and what affects it.   22

2.6
Distribution of drug
resistant malaria.   23

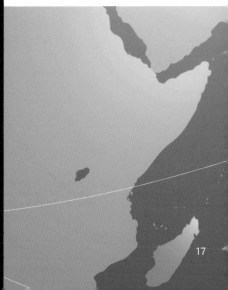

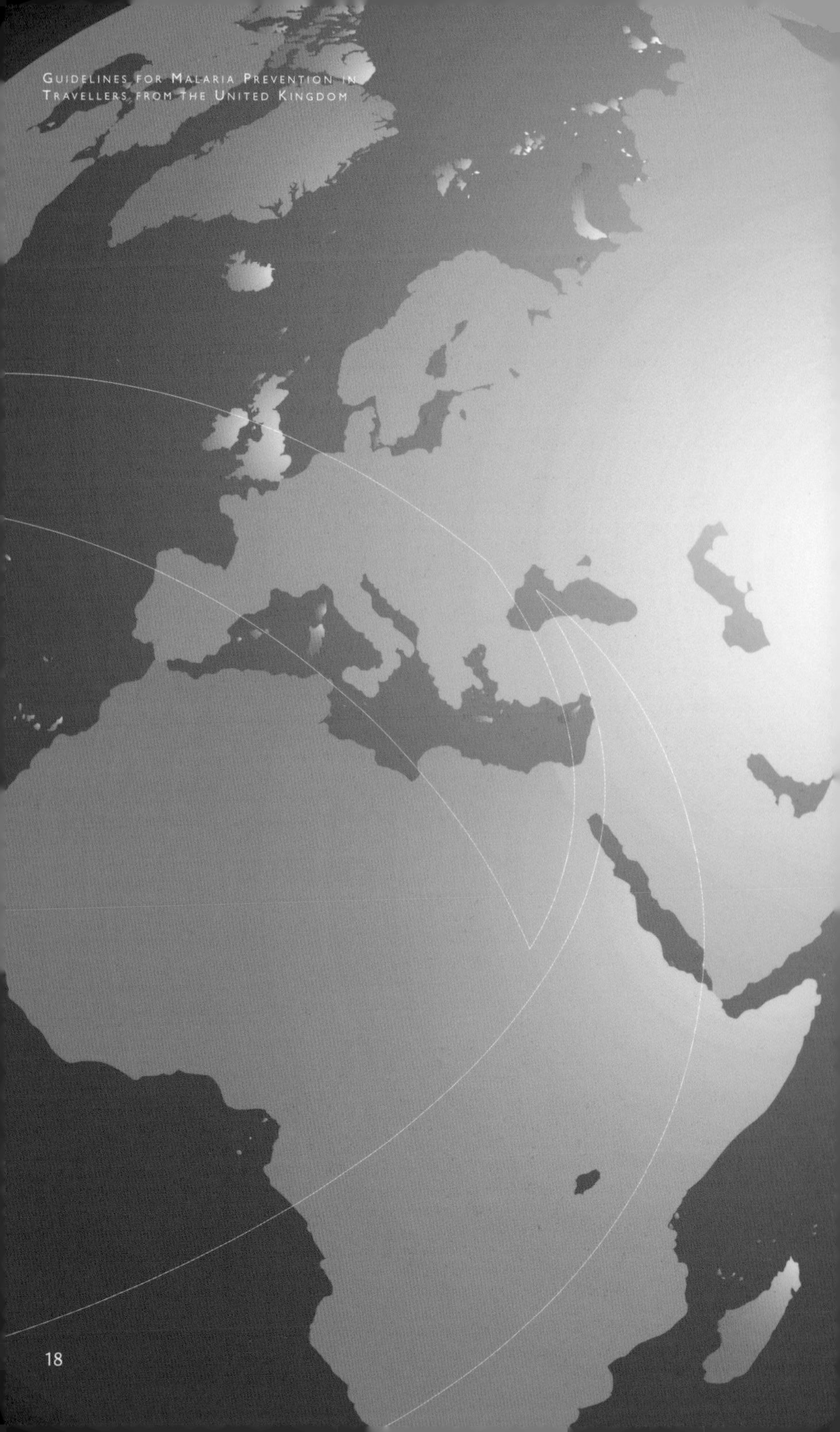

2. Awareness of Risk

2.1 What is malaria?

Malaria is a serious febrile illness due to infection of red blood cells with a parasite called *Plasmodium*. It is transmitted by mosquitoes.

Four species of *Plasmodium* commonly infect humans; see table 1 below.

TABLE 1	PLASMODIUM SPECIES WHICH INFECT HUMANS	
SPECIES	**COMMENT**	**NUMBER OF CASES REPORTED IN THE UK IN 2005 OUT OF 1754**
Plasmodium falciparum	The most dangerous, responsible for the vast majority of malaria deaths worldwide	1338 (76%)
Plasmodium vivax	A relapsing malaria See life cycle	258 (15%)
Plasmodium ovale	A relapsing malaria See life cycle	116 (7%)
Plasmodium malariae	The species least commonly seen in the UK. May present with late recrudescence after many years	29 (2%)

Mixed infections with more than one species of malaria parasite are not commonly reported (10 in 2005).

FIGURE I | THE MALARIA LIFE CYCLE

The places in the life cycle targeted by the various preventative measures are shown.

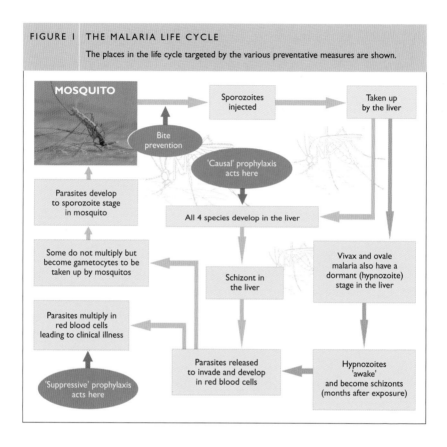

2.2 Life cycle

An infected mosquito inoculates 10 to 15 sporozoites when it bites. Each sporozoite introduced into a human and successfully entering a liver cell develops in the case of *P. falciparum* in five to seven days into a schizont containing approximately 30,000 offspring (merozoites) which are released into the bloodstream when the schizont ruptures. Each merozoite has the potential to infect a red blood cell. Once inside the red cell, the malaria parasite grows and divides over 48 hours (*P. falciparum, vivax* or *ovale*) to 72 hours (*P. malariae*) to form between 8 and 32 parasites whereupon the red cell bursts to release them to infect new red cells. These cycles in the red cells continue, increasing the numbers of parasites in the infected person and leading to clinical illness. Some parasites in the red cells do not divide but form sexual stages (gametocytes) which mate if taken up by a biting female mosquito and thus complete the malaria life cycle. Figure 1 shows the points in the life cycle at which antimalarial preventive measures are targeted.

2.3 The malarial illness

Malaria can neither be confirmed nor excluded by clinical features alone. The common symptoms and signs are shown in Table 2. There may be no physical signs apart from fever but it must be noted that even the absence of fever itself does not exclude the diagnosis in an ill patient. There is a risk of misdiagnosing malaria as influenza or other viral illness: viral hepatitis (if jaundice is present), gastroenteritis (if diarrhoea is evident) or lower respiratory tract infection (cough can be a non-specific symptom).

TABLE 2   CLINICAL SYMPTOMS AND SIGNS OF MALARIA
(from the ACMP Malaria Treatment Guidelines)

NON-SPECIFIC SYMPTOMS OF MALARIA
Fever/sweats/chills   *Malaise (vague discomfort)*   *Myalgia (muscle pain, tenderness)*   *Headache*   *Diarrhoea*   *Cough*
MAJOR FEATURES OF SEVERE OR COMPLICATED FALCIPARUM MALARIA IN ADULTS
Impaired consciousness or seizures   *Renal impairment (oliguria < 0.4ml/kg bodyweight per hour or creatinine >265µmol/l))*   *Acidosis (pH <7.3)*   *Hypoglycaemia (<2.2mmol/l)*   *Pulmonary oedema or acute respiratory distress syndrome (ARDS)*   *Haemoglobin ≤8g/dL*   *Spontaneous bleeding/disseminated intravascular coagulation*   *Shock (algid malaria)*   *Haemoglobinuria (without G6PD deficiency)*
MAJOR FEATURES OF SEVERE OR COMPLICATED MALARIA IN CHILDREN
Impaired consciousness or seizures   *Respiratory distress or acidosis (pH <7.3)*   *Hypoglycaemia*   *Severe anaemia*   *Prostration (inability to sit or stand)*   *Parasitaemia >2% red blood cells parasitized*

FIGURE 2   GLOBAL DISTRIBUTION OF MALARIA AS ASSESSED BY
THE WORLD HEALTH ORGANIZATION IN 2003

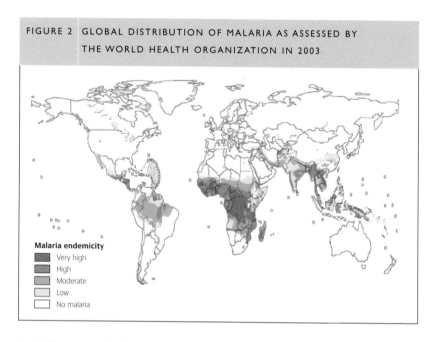

Malaria endemicity
- Very high
- High
- Moderate
- Low
- No malaria

2.4 Where is malaria found?

Figure 2 shows the global distribution of malaria as assessed by the World Health Organization (WHO) in 2003[2].

In-country maps of prophylactic advice linked to malaria distribution are available in the web-based version of these guidelines for use when advising individual travellers. The likelihood of malaria transmission may vary considerably within one country.

2.5 Level of risk of exposure to malaria and what affects it

Exposure of individual travellers to malaria is influenced by the number of infectious bites received. Conditions affecting number of infectious bites received are given below.

Temperature, altitude and season

- The optimum conditions for malaria transmission are high humidity and an ambient temperature in the range 20 to 30°C[3].
- Malaria transmission does not occur in regions with temperatures below the 16°C isotherm (line on a weather map joining all the places that have the same temperature).
- Parasite maturation in the mosquito cannot take place at altitudes greater than 2000 metres.
- Seasonal rainfall increases mosquito breeding.

Rural versus urban location

- Malaria prevalence is generally higher in rural than in urban areas, especially in Africa where the intensity of transmission is on average about 8 times higher in villages than towns[4] but the risk of contracting malaria in African or other cities of malaria-endemic areas must not be discounted[5].

Type of accommodation

- An impregnated bed net should be used unless the accommodation is fitted with functioning air-conditioning and windows and doors which are sufficiently well sealed to prevent mosquito entry.
- Backpackers staying in cheap accommodation have a higher risk of being bitten compared to tourists staying in air-conditioned hotels.
- The traveller should embark on their journey equipped with mosquito protection measures appropriate to their particular circumstances.

Patterns of activity

- Being outdoors between dusk and dawn when *Anopheles* mosquitoes bite increases the risk.

Length of stay

- The longer the stay, the higher the risk of contracting malaria.

2.6 Distribution of drug resistant malaria

- Chloroquine resistant falciparum malaria is now widespread. *P. falciparum* has also developed resistance to a variety of other agents in certain areas. Further comment on the extent and severity of drug resistance is given in tables 7-12 in chapter 4.
- There is currently no recorded drug resistance to *Plasmodium ovale* and only one report of drug-resistant *P. malariae* (to chloroquine)[6].

- Chloroquine-resistant *P. vivax* is found in Papua New Guinea and Irian Jaya; with sporadic reports from elsewhere in Oceania, Asia, South America, Ethiopia and Somalia.
- *P. vivax* with reduced susceptibility to primaquine (the Chesson strain) is found in South-East Asia and Oceania and higher doses of primaquine are required to achieve radical cure of this parasite.

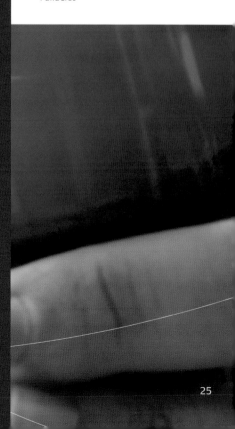

3 - Bite Prevention

3.1
When do female *Anopheles*
mosquitoes bite?   27

3.2
Measures to prevent
mosquito bites.   27
   Repellents
   Insecticides
   Nets
   Clothing
   Room protection
   Fallacies

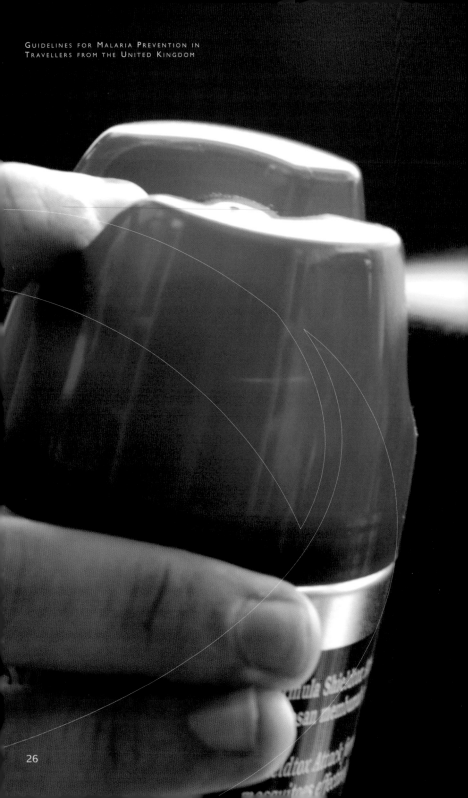

3. Bite Prevention

Effective bite prevention should be the first line of defence against malarial infection.

3.1 When do female Anopheles mosquitoes bite?

Biting time varies between species, so travellers should assume they are at risk of being bitten from dusk to dawn inclusive. The biting of the two main malaria vectors in Africa peaks at about 2am so protection in bed is especially important. As other species of mosquito e.g. those which transmit dengue fever bite during the daytime, it would be prudent to also maintain bite precautions during daylight hours.

3.2 Measures to prevent mosquito bites

3.2.1 Repellents

ACMP strongly recommends DEET-based insect repellents. If DEET is not tolerated (or is not available), an alternative preparation should be used, but few are as effective as DEET (see below).

DEET

DEET (N,N-diethyl-m-toluamide) has been in use as an insect repellent for more than 50 years. It is available in a variety of concentrations and in various preparations including sprays and a slow release polymer.

Duration of protection is 1 to 3 hours for 20%, up to 6 hours for 30% and up to 12 hours for 50% DEET. There is no further increase in duration of protection beyond a concentration of 50%. Sweat-off time varies with activity. The interval between applications depends on this as well as the DEET formulation and concentration used.

When both sunscreen and DEET are required, DEET should be applied afterwards. DEET reduces the efficacy of sunblock, however sunscreens do not reduce the effectiveness of DEET[7,8].

DEET is not recommended for infants below the age of 2 months.

Use of 20% DEET in the second and third trimesters of pregnancy was not associated with adverse effects on infants from those pregnancies followed for up to 12 months after birth[9]. Given the seriousness of malaria in pregnancy, ACMP recommends the use of DEET at a concentration of up to 50% as part of the malaria prevention regimen for pregnant women, including those in the first trimester. DEET may be used at a concentration of up to 50% in breast feeding and for infants and children aged over 2 months.

ACMP advice on use of DEET for protection from mosquito bites:

- DEET is suitable for all individuals over the age of 2 months (unless allergic).
- 50% has the longest duration of action, and needs fewer applications per day.

- There is no evidence that any group (including pregnant women and small children) is at increased risk from using 50% DEET.
- Lower concentrations are available: they need more frequent application and may not be as effective as 50%-care must be taken to re-apply or use a higher concentration DEET preparation if mosquito biting occurs after their use. Lower concentrations are not suitable for individuals who may expect prolonged exposure, such as that encountered by backpackers and expedition travellers.
- ACMP considers concentrations below 20% inappropriate in any circumstances.
- DEET applications can damage some plastic watch straps, watch 'glasses' and plastic jewellery; these items should not be allowed to come into contact with DEET.

p-menthane 3,8 diol (lemon eucalyptus)

p-menthane 3,8 diol (PMD) gives about the same amount of protection afforded by 15% DEET[10] but is reported to provide a shorter period of protection than extended duration (microencapsulated) DEET[11].

Picaridin (Icaridin)

Picaridin (KBR3023) (1-piperidinecarboxylic acid, 2-(2-hydroxyethyl)-,1-methyl-propylester) is reported to have repellent properties comparable to those of DEET[12-14]. Picaridin is sold in Europe as a 20% formulation whilst a 7% picaridin formulation is on sale in the US[15]. If a traveller elects to use picaridin for mosquito bite prevention, ACMP advises use of a 20% preparation.

3-ethlyaminopropionate

3-ethlyaminopropionate (IR3535) has a shorter duration of protection than DEET[13,16].

Oil of Citronella

Whilst oil of citronella-based products do have repellent properties, they provide short-lived protection[16] and are not recommended by ACMP. Citronella has been withdrawn in Europe.

3.2.2 *Insecticides*

Permethrin and other synthetic pyrethroids have a rapid knock-down effect on mosquitoes and are used to kill resting mosquitoes in a room.

3.2.3 Nets

If sleeping outdoors or in unscreened accommodation, insecticide-treated mosquito nets should be used. Protective efficacy for travellers has been estimated at 50%[17].

Mosquito bed nets must be free of tears and should be tucked in under the mattress.

Insecticide (pyrethroid)-impregnated bed nets improve protection because they help to prevent (a) biting through the net on part of the body touching the net, (b) mosquitoes surviving long enough near a net to find any tears in the net which may exist (c) diversion of mosquitoes from someone under a net to someone in the same room without a net[18].

Nets need to be re-impregnated every 6 to 12 months (depending on how frequently the net is washed) to remain effective. If a traveller purchases an impregnated net, the 6 months starts from the date when it starts to be used and washed, as washing and handling are the main factors removing the pyrethroid. Long-lasting nets, in which the pyrethroid is incorporated into the material of the net itself or bound to it with a resin, are now available. These have an expected useful life of 3 to 5 years and are expected to supersede nets which require re-impregnation.

3.2.4 Clothing

Within the limits of practicality, cover up with long-sleeved, loose-fitting clothing, long trousers and socks if out of doors after sunset, to minimise accessibility to skin for biting mosquitoes. There is no evidence that the colour of clothing is relevant to mosquitoes. Clothing may be sprayed or impregnated with permethrin[19] or purchased pre-treated to reduce biting through the clothing. As an alternative, cotton clothing (e.g. socks) can be sprayed with DEET.

3.2.5 Room protection

Air conditioning reduces the likelihood of mosquito bite as a result of substantial reduction in night time temperature. Ceiling fans reduce mosquito nuisance.

Doors, windows and other possible mosquito entry routes to sleeping accommodation should be screened with fine mesh netting which must be close-fitting and free from tears.

The room should be sprayed before dusk with a knockdown insecticide (usually a pyrethroid) to kill any mosquitoes which may have entered the accommodation during the day.

During the night, where electricity is available, use an electrically heated device to vapourise a "mat" (tablet) containing a synthetic pyrethroid in the room. A new mat is needed each night.

Burning of a mosquito coil is an alternative but is not as effective[20] and is not recommended for indoor use.

3.2.6 Fallacies

Herbal remedies

The ACMP strongly advises against relying on any herbal remedies for the prevention of malaria. Herbal remedies have not been tested for their ability to prevent or treat malaria.

Homoeopathy

The ACMP strongly advises against relying on any homoeopathic remedies for the prevention of malaria. There is no scientific proof that homoeopathic remedies are effective in either preventing or treating malaria. In addition, the Faculty of Homeopathy does not promote the use of homoeopathic remedies for disease prevention and notes that their use in malaria prevention is unlikely to be acceptable to insurance providers.

Buzzers

Electronic buzzers (emitting high frequency sound waves) are completely ineffective as mosquito repellents. Companies selling them have been prosecuted and fined under the UK Trades Descriptions Act and ACMP advice is that they should not be used.

Vitamin B1

There is no evidence that vitamin B1 taken orally repels mosquitoes[21,22].

Garlic

There is no evidence that garlic taken orally repels mosquitoes[23].

Savoury yeast extract spread

It is sometimes stated that Marmite® taken orally repels mosquitoes either by giving off a cutaneous odour repellent to mosquitoes or via its vitamin B1 content. There is no evidence that either assertion is true.

Tea tree oil

There is no evidence that tea tree oil is an effective mosquito repellent.

Bath oils

There is no evidence that proprietary bath oils provide effective protection against mosquito bites.

"Once you get malaria it keeps coming back"

Hypnozoite-induced relapses occur in vivax and ovale malaria, but can be treated successfully and further relapses prevented. If the patient has received a full course of treatment with modern antimalarial drugs and has not been re-exposed to malaria, it is extremely unlikely that a history of recurrent febrile illness over a number of years is the result of chronic malaria.

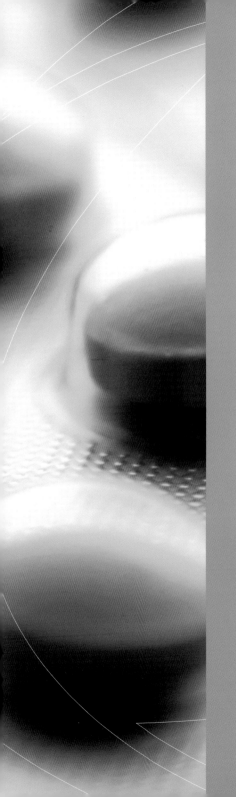

4 - Chemoprophylaxis

4.1
Principles.   33

4.2
The drugs.   34
  Chloroquine
  Proguanil
  Chloroquine plus proguanil
  Mefloquine
  Doxycycline
  Atovaquone plus proguanil

4.3
Dosage tables.   39

4.4
Country tables.   42

4.5
Popular destinations.   53

4.6
Emergency Standby Treatment.   54

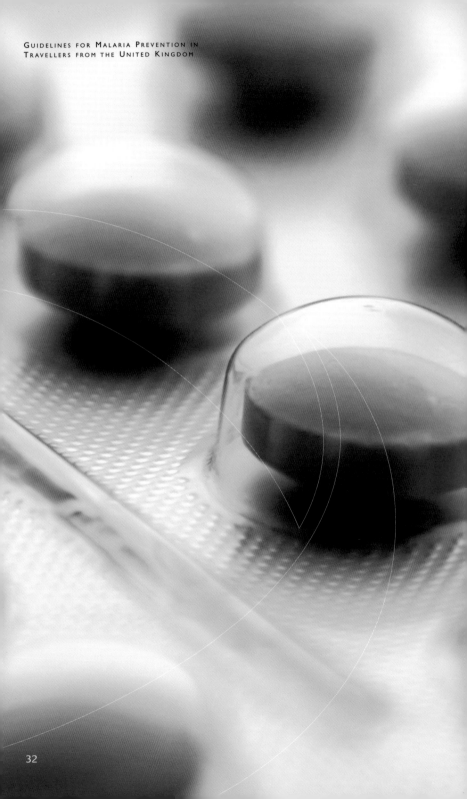

4. Chemoprophylaxis

Given the possibility of antimalarials purchased in the tropics being fake[24], travellers should obtain the medication required for their chemoprophylaxis from a reputable source in the UK before they travel. ACMP also advises against purchasing antimalarial drugs over the internet.

4.1 Principles

Causal prophylaxis

Causal prophylaxis is directed against the liver stage of the malaria parasite, which takes approximately 7 days to develop (see life cycle in figure1). Successful drug activity at this stage prevents the parasite from progressing to infect red blood cells.

Causal prophylactics need to be given for approximately 7 days after infection[25], so ACMP recommends that they are continued for 7 days after leaving a malarious area (see table 3 of drug regimens in chapter 4).

It is important not to confuse liver-stage schizonts with hypnozoites. All 4 species of human malaria have liver-stage schizonts but only *Plasmodium vivax* and *P. ovale* have the hypnozoite stage, against which causal prophylaxis is NOT effective.

Suppressive prophylaxis

Suppressive prophylaxis is directed against the red blood cell stages of the malaria parasite and thus needs to be taken for several weeks to prevent infection[26].

Therefore, suppressive prophylactic drugs should be continued for 4 weeks after leaving a malarious area (see drug regimens in table 3, Chapter 4).

Prophylaxis against hypnozoites

Plasmodium vivax and *P. ovale* have a dormant stage called the "hypnozoite". The hypnozoite remains dormant for months and then "wakes up" to develop into a liver schizont. The dormant hypnozoite explains why attacks of vivax or ovale malaria can occur long after the end of chemoprophylaxis. This is not due to drug failure as none of the prophylactic drugs currently advised by ACMP, acts against the hypnozoite stage of *P. vivax* or *P. ovale*.

Primaquine is active against hypnozoites (present only in *P.vivax* and *P.ovale*) and also has causal prophylactic activity against the liver stage schizonts of all 4 malaria parasites of humans[27]. Primaquine is occasionally used for terminal prophylaxis (also known as presumptive anti-relapse therapy) to eradicate hypnozoites of *P.vivax* and *P.ovale*. However, the routine use of primaquine for prophylaxis is not recommended by ACMP. Practitioners considering the use of primaquine as a prophylactic agent should consult an expert centre (see Chapter 9).

Primaquine is an oxidant drug and can lead to haemolysis in G6PD-deficient individuals.

33

4.2 The drugs

The British National Formulary (BNF) contains full listings of drug actions, dosages, side effects, interactions and contraindications summarised here and should be consulted as required when recommending malaria chemoprophylaxis.

Chapter 6 of this book also provides details of contraindications for different medical conditions such as pregnancy and renal impairment.

NOTE: All adverse events of medication, including attacks of malaria, should be reported. Members of the public and healthcare professionals can report any suspected side effects from malaria medicines via the Yellow Card Scheme on the Medicines and Healthcare products Regulatory Agency (MHRA) website. www.mhra.gov.uk

These drugs are not listed in order of preference.

4.2.1 Chloroquine

Mode of action

Chloroquine is concentrated in the malaria parasite lysosome and is thought to act by interfering with malaria pigment formation, causing generation of a ferriprotoporphyrin IX-chloroquine complex which is highly toxic to the parasite.

Efficacy

Chloroquine-resistant falciparum malaria is now reported from all WHO regions except Central America north of the Panama Canal and the Island of Hispaniola (Haiti & the Dominican Republic). Prophylaxis with chloroquine as a single agent is therefore rarely appropriate (see tables 7-12). It remains effective against most *P. vivax*, all *P. ovale* and virtually all *P. malariae*.

Side-effects

The main side effects are gastrointestinal disturbances and headache. Convulsions are recorded. Chloroquine may cause itching in persons of African descent.

Interactions

Drugs: Amiodarone (increased risk of ventricular arrhythmias); ciclosporin (increased risk of toxicity); digoxin (possibly increases plasma concentration of digoxin); mefloquine (increased risk of convulsions); moxifloxacin (increased risk of ventricular arrhythmias; avoid concomitant use).

Vaccines: Chloroquine may suppress the antibody response to pre-exposure intradermal human diploid cell rabies vaccine[28]. This interaction is not seen when rabies vaccine is given intramuscularly (the currently recommended mode of vaccination in the UK).

Contraindications

Chloroquine prophylaxis may exacerbate psoriasis and myasthenia gravis. It is contraindicated in those with a history of epilepsy.

Cautions

Chloroquine is highly toxic in overdosage, so should be stored out of the reach of children. In long term use, eye examinations every 6-12 months should be considered at 6 years prophylactic usage, though the risk of retinopathy developing on prophylactic dosage is considered to be very low[29]. See also long-term traveller section in chapter 7.

Methods of administration

Tablets contain 155 or 150 mg chloroquine base; syrup contains chloroquine base 50 mg/5 ml (see paediatric dosages in tables 4 and 5). Adult dose 300 mg (2 tablets) weekly, starting one week before entering a malarious area, continuing throughout the time in the area and for 4 weeks after leaving the area.

4.2.2 Proguanil

Mode of action

Proguanil is converted to an active metabolite cycloguanil which inhibits the enzyme dihydrofolate reductase and interferes with the synthesis of folic acid. It acts as a suppressive and also as a causal prophylactic[30]. Proguanil itself has a second mode of action, mediated by the parent drug rather than its metabolite, which produces synergy with atovaquone (see atovaquone plus proguanil).

Efficacy

There are very few regions in the world where the local *Plasmodium falciparum* strains are fully sensitive to proguanil, so prophylaxis with proguanil as a single agent is rarely appropriate (see country tables 7-12, chapter 4).

Side-effects

The principal side effects of proguanil are mild gastric intolerance and diarrhoea. Mouth ulcers and stomatitis occur occasionally, particularly when combined with chloroquine.

Interactions

Drugs: May enhance the anticoagulant effect of warfarin. Absorption reduced by oral magnesium salts. Antifolate effect is increased when given with pyrimethamine.

Vaccines: None reported.

Contraindications

Allergy to proguanil.

Cautions

Renal impairment. Pregnancy (folate supplements required).

Methods of administration

100mg tablets only. Adult dose 200 mg daily, starting one week before entering a malarious area, continuing throughout the time in the area and for 4 weeks after leaving the area.

4.2.3 Chloroquine plus proguanil

For side effects, interactions, contraindications and methods of administration, please see individual agents.

ACMP does not recommend the use of chloroquine plus proguanil for travellers to sub-Saharan Africa. If no alternative is felt to be appropriate, the matter should be discussed with an expert centre (see chapter 9).

4.2.4 Mefloquine

Mode of action

Mefloquine's mode of action has not been determined, but is thought to be unrelated to that of chloroquine and not to involve an anti-folate action. It acts as a suppressive prophylactic.

Efficacy

The protective efficacy of mefloquine is approximately 90% in Africa[31]. At the present time, significant resistance of P. falciparum to mefloquine is a problem only in some areas of south-East Asia[32], but is reported sporadically from the Amazon basin.

Side-effects

Attention has focused on neuropsychiatric problems with mefloquine prophylaxis. Increased moderate problems have been found especially in women using mefloquine when compared with those receiving doxycycline, or atovaquone plus proguanil, but not those taking chloroquine plus proguanil[33] but there is no evidence that mefloquine use increases the risk of first-time diagnosis of depression[34] and no association between mefloquine prescriptions and hospitalisation[35]. Overall, mefloquine remains an important prophylactic agent which is tolerated by the majority of travellers who take it[36].

Interactions

Drugs: Mefloquine antagonises the anticonvulsant effect of antiepileptics and interacts with a number of cardiac drugs.

Contraindications

Mefloquine prophylaxis is contraindicated in those with a current or previous history of depression, neuropsychiatric disorders or epilepsy; or with hypersensitivity to quinine.

Cautions

Pregnancy; (see Chapter 6,special groups) breast-feeding; (see Chapter 6, special groups) cardiac conduction disorders. Not recommended in infants under 3 months (5kg).

Can mefloquine be taken by those who plan to undertake underwater diving?

If the individual tolerates mefloquine prophylaxis, there is no evidence that they cannot physically perform underwater diving. However, it should be noted that some sub-aqua centres do not permit those taking mefloquine to dive.

Although mefloquine may be suitable for scuba divers who have taken and tolerated the drug before, or those able to start taking it early to ensure that no adverse events occur, it should usually be avoided: it lowers the seizure threshold (and may therefore add to the complications of decompression or narcosis events) and some neuropsychiatric adverse events, though excessively rare, can be sudden in onset.

Airline pilots

The UK Civil Aviation Authority advises that mefloquine should not be administered to airline pilots, although there is no evidence that mefloquine impairs function.

Methods of administration

Oral. 250mg tablets. Weekly dosage, starting 2-3 weeks before entering a malarious area to assess tolerability, continuing throughout the time in the area and for 4 weeks after leaving the malarious area.

4.2.5 Doxycycline

Mode of action

Doxycycline is lipophilic and acts intracellularly, binding to ribosomal mRNA and inhibiting protein synthesis. It acts as a suppressive prophylactic.

Efficacy

Doxycycline is of comparable prophylactic efficacy to mefloquine[37].

Side-effects

Doxycycline hydrochloride preparations have a low pH and may produce oesophagitis, especially if taken on an empty stomach and/or just before lying down. Rarely, doxycycline may cause photosensitivity which is mostly mild and transient[38]. Doxycycline is a broad spectrum antibiotic and may predispose to vaginal candidiasis.

Interactions

Drugs: The metabolism of doxycycline is accelerated by carbamazepine and phenytoin. At present, there are no data to support a change in the dose of doxycycline used for malaria prophylaxis in individuals taking one or more of these agents. Tetracyclines possibly enhance the anticoagulant effect of coumarins (e.g. warfarin), and may increase plasma concentration of ciclosporin. It may temporarily reduce the contraceptive effect of oestrogens (see FAQs in Chapter 8).

Vaccines: Possibly reduces the efficacy of oral typhoid vaccine if given simultaneously. Should be separated by 24 hours.

Contraindications

Children under 12 years of age. Pregnancy and breast feeding. Allergy to tetracyclines.

Cautions

Hepatic impairment. Patients taking potentially hepatotoxic drugs. Myasthenia gravis. Systemic lupus erythematosus.

Methods of administration

Capsules (50 or 100mg) or dispersible 100mg tablets only (consult summary of product characteristics pertaining to individual products). Dose 100mg daily, starting 1 to 2 days before entering a malarious area, continuing whilst there and for 4 weeks after leaving.

Precautions in use

The prescriber should warn against excessive sun exposure (and advise on the correct use of sunscreen), the risk of vaginal candidiasis and the risk of oesophagitis if taken on an empty stomach and/or lying down too soon after taking it. Doxycycline should be swallowed whole with plenty of fluid during meals while sitting or standing.

4.2.6 Atovaquone plus proguanil (Malarone®)

Mode of action

Atovaquone works by inhibiting electron transport in the mitochondrial cytochrome b-c1 complex, causing collapse in the mitochondrial membrane potential. This action is potentiated by proguanil and is not dependent upon conversion to its metabolite cycloguanil. Indeed, the combination remains effective in cycloguanil-resistant parasites[39]. Atovaquone/proguanil prevents development of pre-erythrocytic (liver) schizonts (but not hypnozoites). It acts as a causal prophylactic agent, so needs to be continued for only 7 days after leaving a malarial area[40]. It also has activity against the erythrocytic stages of malaria parasites and is useful for treatment.

Efficacy

Prophylactic efficacy against P. falciparum is in excess of 90%[41-48]. There is less published data on protection against P. vivax, but data available indicate that atovaquone-proguanil is effective in the prevention of primary attacks of vivax malaria[44,49]. However, like chloroquine-proguanil, mefloquine and doxycycline, it will not protect against hypnozoite-induced episodes of P.vivax (or P.ovale) malaria.

Side-effects

The most frequent side-effects are headache and gastrointestinal upsets.

Interactions

For proguanil see proguanil section (above).

Drugs: Plasma concentration of atovaquone is reduced by rifabutin and rifampicin (possible therapeutic failure of atovaquone), tetracycline (clinical significance of this is not known) and metoclopramide.

Antiretrovirals: Atovaquone possibly reduces plasma concentration of indinavir. Atovaquone possibly inhibits metabolism of zidovudine (increased plasma concentration).

Vaccines: None reported.

Contraindications

Pregnancy: The BNF states "Manufacturer advises avoid unless essential." ACMP advises against the use of atovaquone/proguanil for antimalarial chemoprophylaxis in pregnancy. Inadvertent conception when using atovaquone/proguanil is not an indication to consider termination of the pregnancy, as no evidence of harm has emerged in data so far available.

Atovaquone/proguanil should generally be avoided in breast feeding, but ACMP advises that atovaquone/proguanil can be used when breast-feeding if there is no suitable alternative antimalarial.

Cautions

Renal impairment (See also the renal impairment section in chapter 6), diarrhoea or vomiting (reduced absorption of atovaquone).

Methods of administration

Tablets containing proguanil 100 mg and atovaquone 250 mg. Paediatric tablets containing proguanil 25 mg and atovaquone 62.5 mg. Adult dose one tablet daily starting 1 to 2 days before entering a malaria endemic area, continuing throughout the time there and for 1 week after leaving. Paediatric dosage given in table 6.

4.3 Dosage tables

TABLE 3   PROPHYLACTIC REGIMENS AGAINST MALARIA IN ADULTS

REGIMEN	DOSE FOR CHEMOPROPHYLAXIS	USUAL AMOUNT PER TABLET (mg)
Areas of chloroquine resistant *P. falciparum*		
Mefloquine	1 tablet weekly	250
Doxycycline	1 tablet/capsule daily	100
Atovaquone-proguanil	1 tablet daily	250 (atovaquone) plus 100(proguanil)
Areas of little chloroquine resistance; poorly effective where extensive resistance		
Chloroquine plus proguanil	2 tablets weekly plus 2 tablets daily	150 (base) 100
Areas without drug resistance		
Chloroquine	2 tablets weekly	150 (base)
Proguanil	2 tablets daily	100

TABLE 4   DOSES OF PROPHYLACTIC ANTIMALARIALS FOR CHILDREN

WEIGHT IN KG	DRUG AND TABLET SIZE				AGE
	CHLOROQUINE 150mg	PROGUANIL 100mg	MEFLOQUINE 250mg	DOXYCYCLINE 100mg	
Under 6.0	0.125 dose 1/4 tablet	0.125 dose 1/4 tablet	Not recommended*	Not recommended	Term to 12 weeks
6.0 to 9.9	0.25 dose 1/2 tablet	0.25 dose 1/2 tablet	0.25 dose 1/4 tablet	Not recommended	3 months to 11 months
10.0 to 15.9	0.375 dose 3/4 tablet	0.375 dose 3/4 tablet	0.25 dose** 1/4 tablet	Not recommended	1 year to 3 yrs 11 months
16.0 to 24.9	0.5 dose 1 tablet	0.5 dose 1 tablet	0.5 dose 1/2 tablet	Not recommended	4 years to 7 yrs 11 months
25.0 to 44.9	0.75 dose 1 1/2 tablets	0.75 dose 1 1/2 tablets	0.75 dose 3/4 tablet	adult dose from age 12y 1 tablet†	8 years to 12 yrs 11 months
45 kg & over	Adult dose 2 tablets	Adult dose 2 tablets	Adult dose 1 tablet	Adult dose 1 tablet	13 years and over

Weight is a better guide than age for children over 6 months, so children should be weighed for the purpose of dosage calculation. Doxycycline is unsuitable for children under 12 years. Caution: In other countries tablet strength may vary.
- The SPC for mefloquine indicates that it can be used for those weighing more than 5 kgs. Therefore, mefloquine (0.25 dose, 1/4 tablet) may be advised for children weighing 5 to 9.9 kg.

*For mefloquine at this age/weight, 0.375 dose would be preferable, but cannot be safely provided by breaking the adult tablet.
†The adult dose is necessary when doxycycline is only available in capsule form and 3/4 is not feasible.
N.B. Atovaquone/proguanil paediatric dosage is given in Table 6.

TABLE 5	TABLE OF DOSES BY SPOON OR SYRINGE* MEASURES FOR CHLOROQUINE SYRUP

WEIGHT IN kg	NUMBER OF 5ML MEASURES (THERE IS OFTEN A HALF SIZE MEASURE AT THE OTHER END OF THE SPOON)	PROPORTION OF ADULT DOSE	AGE
Under 4.5 kg	0.5 (2.5 ml)	0.083	Under 6 weeks
4.5 - 7.9	1.0 (5.0 ml)	0.167	6 weeks - 5 months
8.0 - 10.9	1.5 (2.5 ml plus 5 ml)	0.250	6 months - 12 months
11.0 - 14.9	2.0 (2 × 5 ml)	0.333	13 months - 2yrs 11 mths
15.0 - 16.5	2.5 (2.5 ml plus2 × 5 ml)	0.417	3 years - 3 yrs 11 mths

N.B. These dose-steps are not the same as for chloroquine tablets, which differ from the syrup in chloroquine content. Chloroquine syrup (Nivaquine ®) contains 50mg chloroquine base in 5ml.
* Chemists may dispense dosing syringes for child doses.

TABLE 6	TABLE OF PAEDIATRIC DOSE OF ATOVAQUONE / PROGUANIL

WEIGHT IN kg	PROPORTION OF ADULT DOSE	NUMBER OF PAEDIATRIC TABLETS
Under 11	Do not use	Not recommended
11 – 20	0.25	1 paediatric
21 – 30	0.50	2 paediatric
31 – 40	0.75	3 paediatric
Over 40	1.00	4 paediatric or 1 adult

4.4 Country tables

TABLE 7	MALARIA CHEMOPROPHYLAXIS IN NORTH AFRICA, THE MIDDLE EAST AND CENTRAL ASIA			
RISK	COUNTRY	ACMP RECOMMENDED REGIMEN	ALTERNATIVE REGIMEN IF RECOMMENDED REGIMEN UNSUITABLE
Risk variable Chloroquine resistance present	Afghanistan (below 2000m, May-November) Iran (rural SE provinces, March-November) Oman (remote rural areas only) Saudi Arabia (risk only in south-western region and in certain rural areas of the Western Region. No risk in Mecca or Medina cities, Jeddah and the high-altitude areas of Asir Province) Tajikistan (June-Oct. especially south border areas) Yemen (no risk in Sana'a city)	Chloroquine plus proguanil	
Risk low	Armenia (June-October) Azerbaijan (southern border area, June-September) Iran (northern border with Azerbaijan, May-October) Egypt (El Faiyum only, June-October) Iraq (rural north in May-November) Syria (north border, May-October) Kyrgystan (South West, May -October) Turkey (Turkey/Syria border plain around Adana and east of there, March-November) Turkmenistan (June-October in South East only)	Chloroquine	Proguanil
Risk very low	Algeria (tiny remote focus) Egypt (whole country is very low risk except El Faiyum areas only) Georgia (some South East villages, July-October) Kyrgystan (except South West- see above) Libya Morocco (few rural areas only) Turkey (most tourist areas) Uzbekistan (sporadic cases in extreme South East only)	Awareness*	

See tables 3-6 for details of regimens

*Awareness of small risk of malaria; avoid mosquito bites and seek medical attention for any suspicious symptoms (up to about a year later) but tablets not considered necessary.

TABLE 8 MALARIA CHEMOPROPHYLAXIS IN SUB-SAHARAN AFRICA

RISK	COUNTRY	ACMP RECOMMENDED REGIMEN	ALTERNATIVE REGIMEN IF RECOMMENDED REGIMEN UNSUITABLE
Risk high Chloroquine resistance widespread	Angola · Benin · Burkina Faso · Burundi · Cameroon · Central African Republic · Chad · Comoros · Congo · Djibouti · Equatorial Guinea · Eritrea · Gabon · Gambia · Ghana · Guinea · Guinea-Bissau · Ivory Coast · Kenya · Liberia · Madagascar · Malawi · Mali · Mozambique · Niger · Nigeria · Principe · Rwanda · São Tomé · Senegal · Sierra Leone · Somalia · Sudan · Swaziland · Tanzania · Togo · Uganda · Zaire · Zambia	Mefloquine OR Doxycycline OR Atovaquone/ Proguanil	Seek expert advice (see chapter 9)
	Botswana (only in the northern half of the country, November-June) Ethiopia (below 2000m, no risk in Addis Ababa) Mauritania (year round in the south; in north July-October) Namibia (northern third only, November-June; all year along Kavango & Kunene Rivers) South Africa (north east, low altitude areas of Mpumalanga & Northern Provinces, including the Kruger National Park, North East KwaZulu-Natal as far south as Tugela River). Zimbabwe (areas below 1200m, November-June; all year in Zambezi valley. Risk negligible in Harare or Bulawayo)		
Risk low	Cape Verde (some risk on São Tiago) Mauritius	Awareness*	

See tables 3-6 for details of regimens
*Awareness of small risk of malaria; avoid mosquito bites and seek medical attention for any suspicious symptoms (up to about a year later) but tablets not considered necessary.

TABLE 9   MALARIA CHEMOPROPHYLAXIS IN SOUTH ASIA

RISK	COUNTRY	ACMP RECOMMENDED REGIMEN	ALTERNATIVE REGIMEN IF RECOMMENDED REGIMEN UNSUITABLE
Risk high Chloroquine resistance high	Bangladesh (only in Chittagong Hill Tract Districts) India (Assam)	Mefloquine OR Doxycycline OR Atovaquone/ Proguanil	Chloroquine plus proguanil
Risk variable Chloroquine resistance usually moderate	Bhutan (southern districts only) India (except for Assam where high risk, and for areas listed below where low risk) Nepal (below 1500m, especially Terai districts; no risk in Kathmandu) Pakistan (below 2000m) Sri Lanka (risk north of Vavuniya)	Chloroquine plus proguanil	Mefloquine OR Doxycycline OR Atovaquone/ Proguanil
Risk low	Bangladesh (except Chittagong Hill Tracts, see above). India (low risk in Southern states of Kerala;Tamil Nadu; Karnataka; Goa and Southern Andhra Pradesh including Hyderabad, and the city of Mumbai (Bombay). Low to no risk in Rajasthan; Uttar Pradesh; Haryana; Punjab; Delhi; Uttaranchal; Himachal Predesh; Jammu & Kashmir. For other areas see above. Sri Lanka (low risk in all areas except north of Vavuniya, see above)	Awareness*	

See tables 3-6 for details of regimens
*Awareness of small risk of malaria; avoid mosquito bites and seek
medical attention for any suspicious symptoms (up to about a year
later) but tablets not considered necessary.

FIGURE 3   INDIA SHOWING THE STATES WITH APPROPRIATE CHEMOPROPHYLAXIS RECOMMENDED

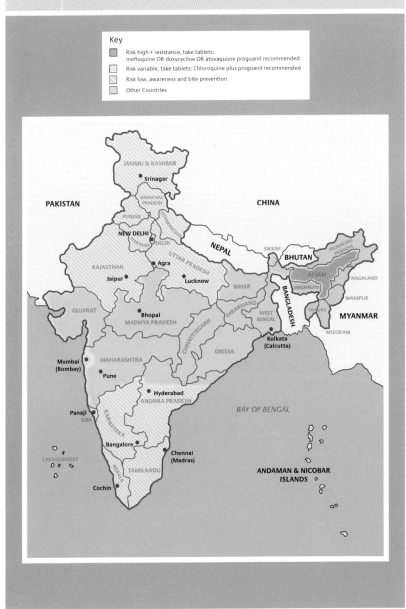

Key

Risk high + resistance, take tablets:
mefloquine OR doxycycline OR atovaquone proguanil recommended

Risk variable, take tablets: Chloroquine plus proguanil recommended

Risk low, awareness and bite prevention

Other Countries

FIGURE 4 BANGLADESH SHOWING THE AREA WHERE CHEMOPROPHYLAXIS RECOMMENDED

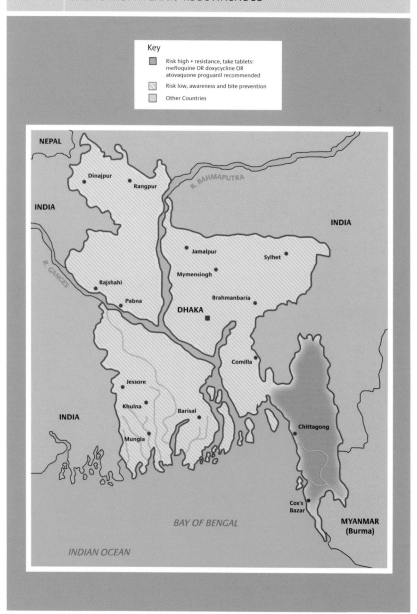

Key

- Risk high + resistance, take tablets: mefloquine OR doxycycline OR atovaquone proguanil recommended
- Risk low, awareness and bite prevention
- Other Countries

FIGURE 5 SRI LANKA SHOWING THE AREA WHERE CHEMOPROPHYLAXIS RECOMMENDED

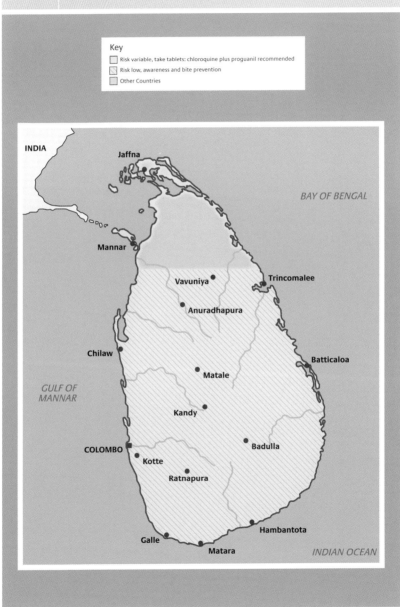

Key
- Risk variable, take tablets: chloroquine plus proguanil recommended
- Risk low, awareness and bite prevention
- Other Countries

TABLE 10 MALARIA CHEMOPROPHYLAXIS IN SOUTH EAST ASIA

RISK	COUNTRY	ACMP RECOMMENDED REGIMEN
Risk high Widespread chloroquine AND mefloquine resistance	Cambodia (western provinces) Thailand (near mainland borders with Cambodia, Laos and Myanmar; low risk and bite avoidance only Chiang Rai and Kwai bridge) Myanmar (eastern part of Shan State)	Doxycycline OR Atovaquone/ Proguanil
Risk high Chloroquine resistance common	Cambodia (except no risk in Phnom Penh) China (only in Yunnan and Hainan; chloroquine in other remote areas of China) East Timor (= Timor-Leste) Papua (Irian Jaya) (part of Indonesia) Laos (except no risk in Vientiane) Lombok (part of Indonesia) Myanmar (formerly Burma [see above for Shan State]) Malaysia East (Sabah only except Kota Kinabalu where awareness and bite prevention advised) Vietnam (except areas listed below that are low risk)	Mefloquine OR Doxycycline OR Atovaquone/ Proguanil
Risk variable Some chloroquine resistance	Indonesia (except Bali and cities where low risk; for Papua (Irian Jaya) and Lombok mefloquine or doxycycline or atovaquone-proguanil recommended) Philippines (rural below 600m; no risk in cities, nor Cebu, Bohol and Catanduanes) Malaysia West (peninsular) Inland forested areas (not Cameron Highlands) and Malaysia East (inland forested areas of Sarawak)	Chloroquine plus proguanil
Risk very low	Bali (part of Indonesia) Brunei China (main tourist areas including Yangtze cruises) Hong Kong Malaysia East (except Sabah (see above) and Sarawak (chloroquine plus proguanil) Malaysia West (low risk including Cameron Highlands except inland forested areas where chloroquine plus proguanil) North Korea (a few southern areas have limited risk) South Korea (limited risk in extreme Northwest) Singapore Thailand (prophylaxis only advised for areas listed above) Vietnam (see above for high risk areas; low risk in cities, coast between Ho Chi Minh and Hanoi, and the Mekong River until close to the Cambodian border)	Awareness*

See tables 3-6 for details of regimens
*Awareness of small risk of malaria; avoid mosquito bites and seek medical attention for any suspicious symptoms (up to about a year later) but tablets not considered necessary.

TABLE 11 MALARIA CHEMOPROPHYLAXIS IN OCEANIA

RISK	COUNTRY	ACMP RECOMMENDED REGIMEN	ALTERNATIVE REGIMEN IF RECOMMENDED REGIMEN UNSUITABLE
Risk high Chloroquine resistance high	Papua New Guinea below 1800m Solomon Islands Vanuatu	Doxycycline OR Mefloquine OR Atovaquone/ Proguanil	Chloroquine plus proguanil (Limited protection)

See tables 3-6 for details of regimens

TABLE 12 MALARIA CHEMOPROPHYLAXIS IN SOUTH AMERICA AND CARIBBEAN

RISK	COUNTRY	ACMP RECOMMENDED REGIMEN	ALTERNATIVE REGIMEN IF RECOMMENDED REGIMEN UNSUITABLE
Risk high Marked chloroquine resistance present	Bolivia (Amazon basin area) Brazil (Amazon basin (i.e. 'Legal Amazon' area, see map); elsewhere very low risk and no chemoprophylaxis) Colombia (most areas below 800m) Ecuador (Esmeraldas Province; see below for elsewhere) French Guiana (especially border areas) Guyana (all interior regions, lesser risk at coast) Peru (Amazon basin area) Suriname (except Paramaribo and coast) Venezuela (all areas south of and including the Orinoco river; north of the river chloroquine plus proguanil recommended see below) Amazon basin areas of Bolivia and Venezuela and Peru	Mefloquine OR Doxycycline OR Atovaquone/ Proguanil	Chloroquine plus proguanil
Risk variable or high Chloroquine resistance present	Bolivia (rural areas below 2500m) Ecuador (areas below 1500m; no malaria in Galapagos Islands nor Guayaquil) Panama (east of canal, canal zone itself no risk) Peru (Other rural areas East of the Andes and West of the Amazon Basin below 1500m) Venezuela (north of the Orinoco river; Caracas free of malaria; south and including Orinoco river, risk high see above)	Chloroquine plus proguanil	Mefloquine OR Doxcycline OR Atovaquone/ Proguanil
Risk variable to low No chloroquine resistance present	Argentina (rural areas along northern borders only) Belize (rural except Belize district) Costa Rica (rural below 500m) Dominican Republic El Salvador (only Santa Ana province in west) Guatemala (below 1500m) Haiti Honduras Mexico (in states of Oaxaca & Chiapas) Nicaragua Panama (west of canal, canal zone itself no risk) Paraguay (some rural areas)	Chloroquine	Proguanil

See tables 3-6 for details of regimens

FIGURE 6 MAP OF AMAZON BASIN AREA SHOWING SPREAD ACROSS SEVERAL SOUTH AMERICAN COUNTRIES

Consult table 12 and figure 7 for details of prophylaxis advised for individual countries.

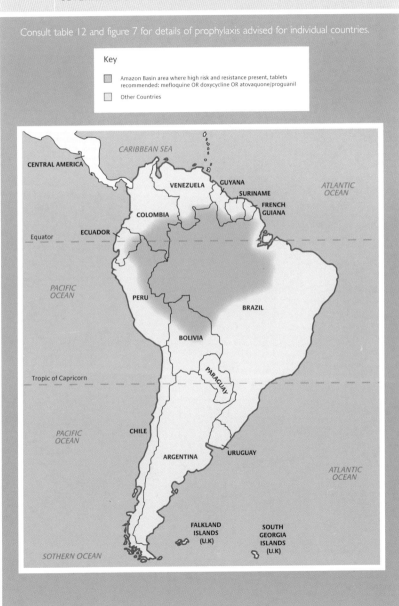

Key

Amazon Basin area where high risk and resistance present, tablets recommended: mefloquine OR doxycycline OR atovaquone/proguanil

Other Countries

FIGURE 7 MAP OF BRAZIL SHOWING THE STATES WHERE CHEMOPROPHYLAXIS IS REQUIRED

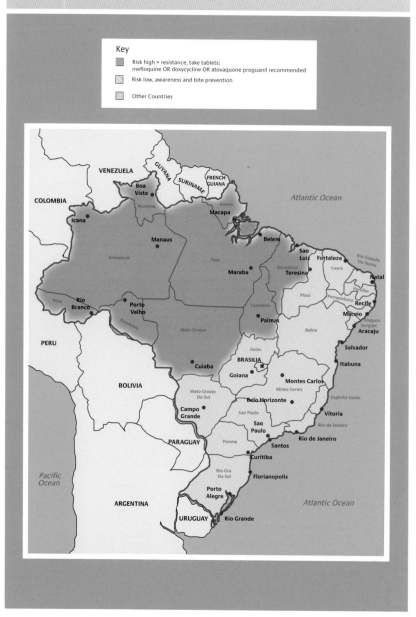

4.5 Popular destinations

TABLE 13 MALARIA CHEMOPROPHYLAXIS FOR POPULAR TOURIST DESTINATIONS

POPULAR DESTINATION	ACMP RECOMMENDED REGIMEN
Angel Falls	Doxycycline OR Mefloquine OR Atovaquone/Proganil
Angkor Wat	Doxycycline OR Mefloquine OR Atovaquone/Proganil
Bali	Awareness*
Chiang Rai	Awareness*
Galapagos Islands	Minimal risk
Goa	Awareness*
Iguacu Falls	Awareness*
Kwai Bridge	Awareness*
Mekong Delta	Awareness*, unless close to the Cambodia border when Mefloquine OR Doxycycline OR Atovaquone/ Proguanil
Turkey (south coast)	Awareness* in tourist resorts, for Adana and the far eastern area: chloroqine

* awareness of small risk of malaria; avoid mosquito bites and seek medical attention for any suspicious symptoms (up to about a year later) but tablets not considered necessary.

4.6 Emergency Standby Treatment

Emergency standby treatment should be recommended for those taking chemoprophylaxis and visiting remote areas where they are unlikely to be within 24 hours of medical attention.

It is intended for those travellers who believe that they may have malaria and is not a replacement for chemoprophylaxis.

It is particularly important that the individual traveller is sufficiently well briefed to be able to use standby emergency treatment appropriately, so written instructions for its use are required, not least because studies from outside the UK have reported standby treatment often being used inappropriately[50].

Standby emergency treatment should be started if it is impossible to consult a doctor and/or reach a diagnosis within 24 hours of the onset of fever.

Medical attention should be sought as soon as possible for full assessment and to exclude other serious causes of fever. This is particularly important as many illnesses other than malaria may present with fever.

The traveller should complete the standby treatment course and recommence their antimalarial chemoprophylaxis 1 week after taking the *first* treatment dose, except in the case of mefloquine prophylaxis, which should be resumed 1 week after the last treatment dose if quinine was used for standby treatment. Antipyretics should be used to treat fever. A second full treatment dose of the antimalarial should be taken if vomiting occurs within 30 minutes of taking it (half-dose if vomiting occurs after 30–60 minutes)[51].

The agent used for emergency standby treatment should be different from the drugs used for chemoprophylaxis, both to minimise drug toxicity and due to concerns over drug resistance[51].

Individuals for whom emergency standby treatment is advised must be provided with written instructions for its use. In particular, they must be informed about symptoms suggesting possible malaria, including fever of 38°C and above, indications for starting the standby treatment, how to take it, expected side-effects and the possibility of drug failure[51].

ACMP recommended regimens for emergency standby treatment are given in table 14.

Specifically, sulfadoxine/pyrimethamine (SP) is NOT recommended due to reports of widespread resistance to this agent among *P. falciparum* strains. Halofantrine is no longer recommended due to concerns over its association with sometimes fatal cardiac arrhythmias[52].

ACMP advises against purchasing antimalarial drugs over the internet.

Antimalarials purchased in the tropics may be fake[24] and travellers should obtain the medication required for their emergency standby treatment from a reputable source in the UK before they travel.

TABLE 14 EMERGENCY STANDBY TREATMENT FOR ADULTS

SITUATION FOR USE	STANDBY TREATMENT REGIMEN	USUAL AMOUNT PER TABLET	ADULT DOSE
Chloroquine or Multi-drug resistant falciparum malaria	Co-artemether (Riamet)	20 mg artemether plus 120 mg lumefantrine	4 tablets initially, followed by 5 further doses of 4 tablets each given at 8, 24, 36, 48 and 60 hours. Total 24 tablets over a period of 60 hours Tablets should be taken with food to enhance drug absorption
Chloroquine or Multi-drug resistant falciparum malaria	Atovaquone plus Proguanil	250 mg plus 100 mg	4 tablets as a single dose on each of three consecutive days
Chloroquine or Multi-drug resistant falciparum malaria	Quinine plus Doxycycline	300 mg quinine and100 mg doxycycline	Quinine 2 tablets 3 times a day for 3 days, accompanied by 1 tablet of doxycycline twice daily for 7 days
Recommended where no chloroquine resistance present NB Now applies to very few geographical areas	Chloroquine (Nivaquine / Avloclor)	150 mg chloroquine base (Nivaquine) or 155 mg chloroquine base (Avloclor)	4 tablets on days 1 & 2, 2 tablets on day 3
Pregnancy	Quinine plus Clindamycin	300 mg quinine 75 or 150 mg (150 mg preferred) clindamycin	Quinine 2 tablets 3 times a day for 5-7 days Clindamycin 3 tablets (450 mg) 3 times a day for 5 days

Chloroquine doses are given as the base.
Quinine plus clindamycin (or chloroquine alone in the very few non-resistant areas) is the only regimen to be used in pregnancy.

Emergency Standby Medication
Traveller Information Leaflet
Available to download from the HPA website www.hpa.org.uk

You have been advised to carry emergency standby antimalarial medication with you on your forthcoming trip. This leaflet provides you with advice on when and how to use it. Please keep it safely with your medication. If you are travelling with a companion, please ask them to read this leaflet as they may be able to assist you in following its advice in the event of your becoming ill.

Incubation period of malaria
The minimum period between being bitten by an infected mosquito and developing symptoms of malaria is 8 days, so a febrile illness starting within the first week of your arrival in a malarious area is not likely to be due to malaria.

Symptoms and signs of malaria
Malaria usually begins with a fever. You may then feel cold, shivery, shaky and very sweaty. Headache, feeling sick and vomiting are common with malaria and you are also likely to experience aching muscles. Some people develop jaundice (yellowness of the whites of the eyes and the skin). It is not necessary for all these symptoms to be present before suspecting malaria as fever alone may be present at first.

When to take your Emergency Standby Medication
If you develop a fever of 38°C [100°F] or more, more than one week after being in a malarious area, please seek medical attention straight away.

If you will not be able to get medical attention within 24 hours of your fever starting, start your standby medication and set off to find and consult a doctor.

How to take your Emergency Standby Medication

First, take medication (usually paracetamol) to lower your fever. If your fever is controlled, it makes it less likely that you will vomit your antimalarial drugs.

Then, without delay, take the first dose of your emergency standby antimalarial medication.

If you do vomit and it is within 30 minutes of taking the antimalarial drugs, repeat the first dose of them (but do not repeat the paracetamol). If you vomit 30–60 minutes after taking the first dose of the antimalarial drugs, repeat the treatment, but take only HALF the first dose.

Continue the treatment as instructed for the particular drugs prescribed for you.

Please remember that this emergency standby medication has been prescribed based on your particular medical history and should be taken only by you as it may not be suitable for others.

Once you have completed your emergency standby medication you should restart your malaria prophylactic drug(s) one week after you took the first treatment dose of. emergency standby medication. If your preventive medication consists of mefloquine and your standby treatment included quinine, you should wait a week *after completing* the course of quinine before you restart mefloquine.

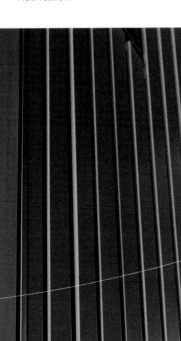

5 - Diagnosis

5.1
Blood tests and how
to request them.   61

5.2
Rapid Diagnostic Tests (RDTs).   61

5.3
Blood film negative malaria.   62

5.4
Resources for treatment advice.   62

5.5
Notification.   62

emergency

5. Diagnosis

Suspected malaria is a medical emergency.

Consider malaria in every ill patient who has returned from the tropics in the previous year, especially in the previous three months.

Fever on return from the tropics should be considered to be malaria until proven otherwise.

Malaria cannot be diagnosed with certainty by clinical criteria alone. Suspected cases should be investigated by obtaining a blood film diagnosis as a matter of urgency. There is no need to wait for fever spikes before taking blood; this only delays diagnosis and the fever pattern seldom conforms to text book periodicity, especially in the case of *Plasmodium falciparum*.

5.1 Blood tests and how to request them in the UK

An EDTA-anticoagulated venous blood sample should be taken.

The sample should be received in the laboratory within one hour of being taken as falciparum malaria may increase in severity over a few hours and the morphology of malaria parasites in EDTA deteriorates over time, rendering accurate laboratory diagnosis more difficult.

Finger-prick samples smeared directly onto microscope slides at the bedside are sub-optimal for modern diagnosis as the laboratory then has no additional material to make and stain further smears, undertake rapid diagnostic tests (RDTs) or refer for PCR testing.

All laboratories making a diagnosis of malaria should send blood films and a portion of the blood sample on which the diagnosis was made to the HPA Malaria Reference Laboratory (MRL) for confirmation (The MRL webpages are available at http:// www.malaria-reference.co.uk

5.2 Rapid Diagnostic Tests (RDTs)

ACMP does not recommend travellers use Rapid Diagnostic Tests (RDTs) for self diagnosis.

RDTs, sometimes known as "dipsticks", permit the detection of malaria parasites in human blood without microscopy. Used correctly, they can confirm the clinical diagnosis of malaria in places remote from medical attention[53] however there is evidence of travellers being unable to use them correctly and thus failing to detect parasites[54].

RDTs do have a place in the medical kit carried by a doctor or nurse accompanying an expedition to remote malarious regions, provided care is taken to transport and store them correctly and thus prevent deterioration in their performance in the field.

5.3 Blood film negative malaria

One negative blood film does not
exclude a diagnosis of malaria. Where
malaria is suspected blood films should
be examined every 12 to 24 hours for
3 days whilst other diagnoses are also
considered. If all three films are negative
and malaria is still considered a possible
diagnosis, expert advice should be
sought from a specialist in tropical or
infectious diseases. It is particularly
important to seek such advice early in
the care of pregnant patients with
suspected malaria, as the main parasite
biomass may be sequestered in the
placenta such that peripheral blood films
are negative despite the patient having
malaria (see chapter 9 for expert advice
listing).

5.4 Resources for treatment advice

The treatment of malaria is outside the
scope of this document and will be
addressed in ACMP malaria treatment
guidelines. Expert advice on malaria
treatment may be obtained from:

The Hospital for Tropical Diseases
http://www.thehtd.org/

The Liverpool School of
Tropical Medicine
http://www.liv.ac.uk/lstm/

Your local infectious diseases unit

See also the British Infection
Society (BIS) website
http://www.britishinfectionsociety.org/
for a malaria treatment algorithm

5.4 Notification

Malaria is a statutorily notifiable disease.
The clinician caring for the patient must
complete a notification form.

The Malaria Reference Laboratory (MRL)
reporting form (MRL website
www.malaria-reference.co.uk) should also
be completed and should be sent to the
MRL separately or along with referred
specimens.

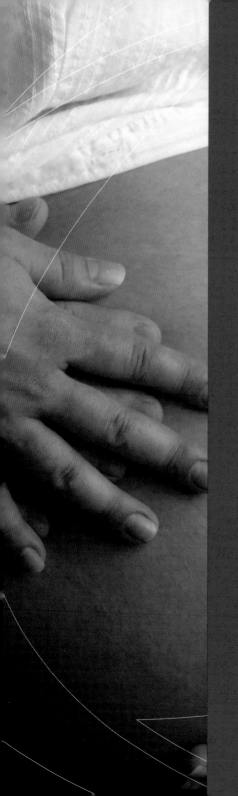

6 - Special Groups
(Medical Conditions)

6.1
Smoking cessation. 65

6.2
Pregnancy. 65

6.3
Breastfeeding. 66

6.4
Anticoagulants. 66

6.5
Epilepsy. 67

6.6
Glucose 6-phosphate
dehydrogenase deficiency. 67

6.7
Sickle Cell disease. 68

6.8
Immunocompromised Travellers. 68
  Risks for transplant patients
  Risks for HIV/AIDS patients

6.9
Liver disease. 69

6.10
Renal impairment. 69

6.11
Splenectomy. 70

6.12
Acute porphyrias. 70

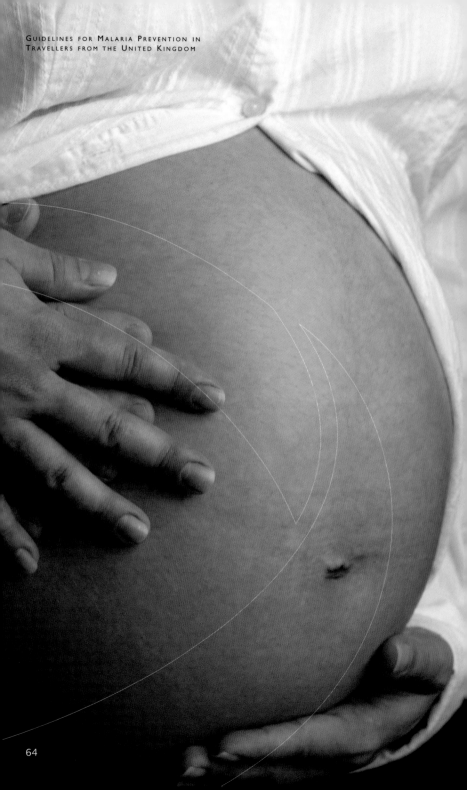

6 Special Groups (Medical Conditions)

6.1 Smoking cessation

Chloroquine or mefloquine should not be used in those taking Zyban® (bupropion hydrochloride SR) as the chances of seizure may be increased.

6.2 Pregnancy

Pregnant women are advised to avoid travel to malarious areas.

In the event that travel is unavoidable, the pregnant traveller must be informed of the risks which malaria presents and the risks and benefits of antimalarial chemoprophylaxis.

Pregnant women have an increased risk of developing severe malaria and a higher risk of fatality compared to non-pregnant women.

Diagnosis of falciparum malaria in pregnancy can be particularly difficult as parasites may not be detectable in blood films due to sequestration in the placenta.

Expert advice is required at an early stage if malaria is suspected in a pregnant woman. Complications, including severe haemolytic anaemia, hypoglycaemia, jaundice, renal failure, hyperpyrexia and pulmonary oedema, may ensue. The result may be miscarriage, premature delivery, maternal and/or neonatal death.

Congenital malaria is rare, but occurs more commonly with *Plasmodium vivax* than with the other malaria parasites of humans.

Avoidance of mosquito bites is extremely important in pregnancy as pregnant women are particularly attractive to mosquitoes. Ideally, pregnant women should remain indoors between dusk and dawn. If they have to be outdoors at night they should adhere rigorously to bite precautions (see chapter 3).

DEET should be used in a concentration of not more than 50%. DEET has a good safety record in children[16] but ingestion should be avoided. Nursing mothers should wash repellents off their hands and breast skin prior to handling infants. See Chapter 3 for further details on DEET.

- Chloroquine and proguanil: safe in all trimesters of pregnancy. Their major disadvantage is the relatively poor protection they give in many geographical areas due to the presence of drug-resistant *P. falciparum*. Pregnant women taking proguanil should receive supplementation with 5 mg folic acid daily.
- Mefloquine: caution advised (see below).
- Doxycycline: contraindicated in pregnancy.
- Atovaquone/proguanil: lack of evidence on safety in pregnancy.

The long-term traveller guidelines[55] describe the evidence for prescribing mefloquine during pregnancy. Briefly, it seems unlikely that mefloquine is associated with adverse foetal outcomes. There is no strong association between mefloquine in treatment doses[56,57], and stillbirths or miscarriages in the second and third trimesters although a lack of data on its use in the first trimester has encouraged caution. The decision whether or not to advise mefloquine prophylaxis in pregnancy therefore requires a careful risk-benefit analysis. Where the levels of transmission and drug resistance (see country tables in chapter 4) make mefloquine an agent of first choice it is generally agreed that mefloquine may be advised in the second and third trimesters of pregnancy. Given the potential severity of falciparum malaria in a pregnant woman, its use may also be justified in the first trimester in areas of high risk of acquiring falciparum malaria such as sub-Saharan Africa, after taking expert advice (see chapter 9).

Women who have taken mefloquine inadvertently just prior to or during the first trimester should be advised that this does not constitute an indication to terminate the pregnancy.

Chemoprophylaxis prior to conception
If a female traveller is planning to conceive during a visit to a destination with a high risk of contracting chloroquine-resistant falciparum malaria, expert advice should be sought (see chapter 9 for advice centres).

Time to allow after finishing a course of an antimalarial before attempting to conceive:
- Mefloquine: 3 months.
- Doxycycline: 1 week.
- Atovaquone/proguanil: 2 weeks.

6.3 Breastfeeding

- Mefloquine: experience suggests safe to use during lactation.
- Doxycycline: contraindicated (do not use).
- Atovaquone/proguanil: not recommended because of the absence of data however, can be used when breast-feeding if there is no suitable alternative antimalarial.

Nursing mothers should be advised to take the usual adult dose of antimalarial appropriate for the country to be visited.

The amount of medication in breast milk will not protect the infant from malaria. Therefore, the breastfeeding child needs his or her own prophylaxis, which for children of breastfeeding age will be either chloroquine plus proguanil or mefloquine. Atovaquone/proguanil may be used if the child weighs 11kg or more.

6.4 Anticoagulants

Travellers who take anticoagulants should ensure their INR (International Normalised Ratio) or clotting time is stable prior to departure.

Patients on warfarin may have underlying cardiovascular disease and may be on cardiovascular medication. Interactions with other medication together with the individuals' medical history should be taken into account when deciding on appropriate malaria chemoprophylaxis.

- Chloroquine: no interaction between warfarin and chloroquine documented in the BNF, although there is a caution in the SPC for Nivaquine.
- Proguanil: an isolated report of an enhanced effect of warfarin when taken together with proguanil[58].
- Mefloquine: not considered to be a problem for those taking warfarin. The manufacturer states that 'although no drug interaction is known with anticoagulants, effects of mefloquine on travellers should be checked before departure.' Please see below for how this can be monitored.
- Doxycycline: the anticoagulant effect of coumarins (including warfarin) is possibly enhanced by tetracyclines[59].
- Atovaquone / proguanil: unknown whether there are interactions between atovaquone/proguanil and warfarin, although there have been isolated reports of an enhanced effect of warfarin when taken together with proguanil (see above under proguanil).

Advice for travellers needing malaria chemoprophylaxis who are taking warfarin:

- Travellers should start taking their malaria tablets more than 1 week (and ideally 2-3 weeks in the case of mefloquine) prior to their departure.
- A baseline INR should be checked prior to starting chemoprophylaxis, and re-checked after 1 week of taking chemoprophylaxis.

- If a traveller is away for a long period of time the INR should be checked at intervals at the destination. (However, the sensitivity of thromboplastin reagent used by some laboratories in different countries may vary[60]).
- Once chemoprophylaxis has been completed, the INR should be checked again to re-stabilise anticoagulant therapy.

6.5 Epilepsy

Proguanil alone (200 mg daily) is recommended for malarious areas without chloroquine resistance. For areas with a high risk of chloroquine-resistant malaria, such as sub-Saharan Africa, doxycycline or atovaquone/proguanil can be used.

- Chloroquine: unsuitable.
- Mefloquine: unsuitable.
- Doxycycline: half-life may be reduced by phenytoin, carbamazepine, and barbiturates, so in theory its dose should be increased for patients taking these drugs. However, there is currently no direct evidence that this is necessary.

6.6 Glucose 6-phosphate dehydrogenase deficiency

Glucose 6-phosphate dehydrogenase (G6PD) is an enzyme that helps protect the red cell against oxidative damage. Absence of G6PD renders the red cell liable to haemolysis in the presence of some drugs.

All G6PD-deficient travellers to malarious areas should take appropriate chemoprophylaxis despite some protection against infection being conferred by the most common G6PD deficiency allele in Africa (G6PD A-)[61].

Chloroquine: theoretical risk of haemolysis in some G6PD-deficient individuals. Haemolysis does not appear to be a problem when chloroquine is given in the dose recommended for malaria chemoprophylaxis so there is no need to withhold chloroquine prophylaxis from those known to be G6PD-deficient. This risk is acceptable in acute malaria[59] and G6PD levels are not usually checked before using chloroquine in treatment doses.

Primaquine: not currently recommended as a first line agent for malaria prevention in UK travellers, but may be considered in special circumstances on expert advice[27]. There is a definite risk of haemolysis in G6PD-deficient individuals. The traveller's G6PD level must be checked before primaquine is prescribed: G6PD deficiency contraindicates its use for prophylaxis.

6.7 Sickle Cell disease

Presence of the sickle cell trait confers some protection against malaria, though individuals with the sickle cell trait still require antimalarial prophylaxis.

For those with homozygous sickle-cell disease, malaria is regarded as a significant cause of morbidity and mortality, producing further haemolysis against the background of that due to sickle-cell disease itself[62]. Therefore, it is essential that individuals with sickle-cell disease travelling to malaria-endemic areas receive rigorous antimalarial protection.

6.8 Immunocompromised travellers

6.8.1 Risks for transplant patients

A review on the prevention of infection in adult travellers after organ transplantation[63] recommended that ciclosporin levels should be monitored if chloroquine is co-administered.

6.8.2 Risks for those with HIV/AIDS

All of the HIV protease inhibitors (PIs) in current use, as well as the non-nucleoside reverse transcriptase inhibitors (NNRTIs) delavirdine and efavirenz, interact with the same liver enzymes which metabolise most drugs used for malaria prophylaxis and treatment. This can result in altered metabolism of antimalarials or antiretrovirals, though the extent of this and the clinical significance is often unclear. The prescriber should check on an individual agent basis.

The extra risk of increased severity if malaria is contracted by an HIV-infected traveller is unclear. Most reported studies have been done in those living in endemic areas where HIV infection increases the risks for contracting and developing severe malaria and increasing immunosuppression reduces treatment success[64] although this varies by area[65]. Co-infected pregnant women are at risk from higher parasite density, anaemia and malarial infection of the placenta. Children born to women with HIV and malaria infection have low birth weight and are more likely to die during infancy. It is unclear whether malaria during pregnancy increases the risk of mother-to-child transmission of HIV[66].

6.9 Liver disease

Most antimalarial drugs are excreted or metabolised by the liver. Thus, there is a risk of drug accumulation in severe liver impairment.

- Severe liver disease: all antimalarial drugs are contraindicated, with the possible exception of atovaquone plus proguanil.
- Moderate impairment: proguanil, or atovaquone plus proguanil or mefloquine may be used.
- Mild impairment: chloroquine, or proguanil, or chloroquine plus proguanil, or atovaquone plus proguanil or mefloquine may be used. Doxycycline should be used only with caution.

The choice of chemoprophylaxis should be made after discussion with the patient's specialist, who will be able to assess their degree of hepatic impairment. The Child-Pugh classification is often used for grading liver function

and can be found at http://www.emea.europa.eu/pdfs/human/ewp/233902en.pdf

6.10 Renal impairment

Chloroquine is partially excreted via the kidneys while proguanil is wholly excreted via the kidneys.

- Chloroquine: dose reduction for prophylaxis is required only in severe renal impairment.
- Proguanil: should be avoided or the dose reduced as shown in table 15. Not to be used in patients receiving renal dialysis.
- Atovaquone/proguanil: not recommended for patients with a creatinine clearance of less than 30mL/minute[59]. Not to be used in patients receiving renal dialysis.

Doxycycline or mefloquine may be used in severe renal failure. There is no need to reduce the dose of mefloquine in renal dialysis[59].

TABLE 15	DOSES OF PROGUANIL IN ADULTS WITH RENAL FAILURE			
	RENAL IMPAIRMENT GRADE	SERUM CREATININE µMOL/LITRE	CREATININE CLEARANCE ML/MIN/1.73M2	PROPHYLACTIC DOSAGE OF PROGUANIL
	(none)	<150	≥ 60	200mg daily (standard dose)
	mild	150-300	20-59	100mg daily
	moderate	300-700	10-19	50mg every second day
	severe	>700	<10	50mg once weekly

6.11 Splenectomy

Those who have no spleen or whose splenic function is severely impaired are at particular risk of severe malaria and, where possible, should avoid travel to malarious areas.

If travel is essential, every effort should be made to avoid infection by rigorous use of antimosquito precautions and strict adherence to appropriate chemoprophyaxis. If the traveller becomes unwell during or after their visit, medical attention is required as a matter of urgency, as malarial parasitaemia in asplenic individuals may rise rapidly to very high levels (e.g. greater than 50% with *P.falciparum*).

6.12 Acute porphyrias

Doxycycline is unsafe in porphyria[59] so should not be used for antimalarial chemoprophylaxis in patients with acute porphyria.

7 - Special Categories

7.1
Children.   73

7.2
Elderly travellers.   74

7.3
Multi-trip travel.   74

7.4
Cruises.   74

7.5
Oil rigs.   75

7.6
Visits to national parks.   75

7.7
Stopovers.   75

7.8
Last minute travellers.   75

7.9
Visiting friends and relatives.   76

7.10
Students and children at
boarding school.   77

7.11
The long-term traveller.   77
Risk Assessment
Chemoprophylaxis for
long-term travellers
Specific considerations
for women
Specific considerations
for infants and older children

7.12
Long term visitors to the UK
returning to live in malarious
parts of the world.   80
Preventive measures
appropriate to an
endemic setting
Prophylaxis

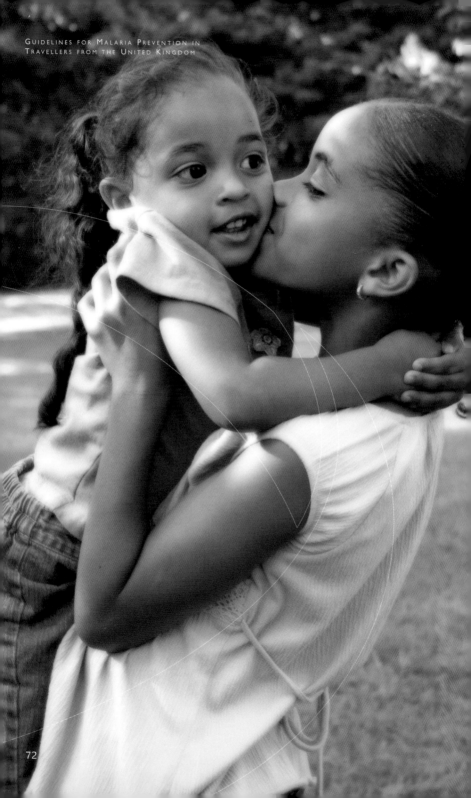

7. Special Categories

7.1 Children

Children are at particular risk of severe and fatal malaria; therefore, parents are advised against taking infants and young children to malarious areas.

If travel is unavoidable, infants and children should be well protected against mosquito bites and receive appropriate malaria chemoprophylaxis.

It is important that the child's carers understand the importance of trying to ensure that the child properly completes the full course of prophylactic medication.

Parents should supervise children's chemoprophylaxis, as some regimens can be difficult even for adults to follow.

Parents must be cautious not to exceed maximum recommended doses, since antimalarials can be particularly toxic to children.

Paediatric doses of antimalarials for prophylaxis are shown in tables 4-6 in chapter 4:

- Chloroquine: Take care to ensure that tablets are actually swallowed, as they have a bitter taste. Sweetened chloroquine syrup is available. Store safely away from children since an overdose can be fatal.

- Proguanil: as for adults more effective when taken with chloroquine although chloroquine resistance is present in many areas. Difficult to use for children since proguanil is only available in adult formulations and, dependent on the weight of the child, the adult-dose tablets must be broken and powdered into food.

- Chloroqine plus proguanil: see individual agents above.

- Mefloquine: Problem in administering correct dosage because there is currently no suspension available and adult-dose tablets must be broken.

- Doxycycline: Only licensed in the UK for children over the age of 12 years due to the bone damaging effects of the drug. This age limit varies between countries; tablets should be swallowed whole and must not be crushed.

- Atovaquone/proguanil: Paediatric tablets are available in the UK for malaria prophylaxis in children from 11 kg upwards. The tablets are a quarter of the strength of adult tablets and can be crushed if necessary for ease of administration.

Whilst it is preferable to avoid breaking and crushing tablets, the appropriate dose of proguanil or mefloquine or atovaquone/proguanil may be crushed if necessary and mixed with jam, honey, chocolate spread or similar food to aid administration to young children. Tablet-cutters can be purchased from some pharmacies or travel shops.

Children with malaria may deteriorate very rapidly to become critically ill. Those looking after children on their return from malarious areas - family members, friends, professional carers, or school nursing and medical staff - should be made aware that such children need medical attention and a blood test for malaria without delay if they become unwell within a year of leaving a malarious area.

Healthcare professionals should strive to improve access to advice on malaria prevention for families with children, especially travellers "Visiting Friends and Relatives".

7.2 Elderly travellers

The elderly are at particular risk from malaria[51]. No reduction in antimalarial dosage is required on the basis of advanced age. However, elderly travellers are more likely to have underlying disorders, for example renal impairment, which may necessitate antimalarial dose reduction. Furthermore, the increased likelihood of elderly travellers taking additional medication, for example for cardiac conditions, will influence the choice of chemoprophylactic agent in their particular case.

7.3 Multi-trip travel

Some travellers, for example business persons or expatriate contract employees, may make several short visits to malarious areas in the same year. For instance someone working in the tropics four weeks on, four weeks off, might be taking chemoprophylaxis for most or all of the year when including the periods before and after travel that prophylaxis is required. The strategy for chemoprophylaxis will then be mainly influenced by the level of malaria risk in the area(s) to be visited. For example, in the highly malarious regions of West Africa, the risk-benefit assessment is strongly in favour of taking chemoprophylaxis, even if it means year-round administration. For less frequent trips, the regions visited should determine the chemoprophylactic agents from which to choose. When the choice lies between mefloquine or doxycycline or atovaquone/proguanil and the traveller wishes tablet-free periods between visits, the shorter period of 7 days post exposure for atovaquone/proguanil prophylaxis versus the alternatives may be helpful.

7.4 Cruises

All travellers on cruises should use insect bite avoidance measures.

Cruises are a growing part of the holiday market. Most travellers on cruises are only ashore during daylight hours when *Anopheles* bites rarely occur, and therefore do not require malaria chemoprophylaxis. However, the cruise itinerary must be reviewed carefully to determine the risk of exposure to malaria.

As examples, cruises in the Caribbean may include several days travelling along the Amazon in Brazil, or Orinoco River in Venezuela. Cruises along the East African coast may include a stop for a night or more in the port of Mombasa, Kenya and passengers may be ashore or on deck after dusk. These itineraries will require malaria chemoprophylaxis.

In addition cruises that have an overnight stay in any other malaria endemic region of the world require malaria chemoprophylaxis.

7.5 Oil rigs

There is a large number of staff employed in the oil industry predominantly based around West Africa. Employees commonly travel to these areas every 4-6 weeks, followed by a similar period of leave back in the UK. Oil rigs may be based in river estuaries or many miles offshore. Thus, the level of risk may be difficult to assess until one period of work has been completed and therefore antimalarial chemoprophylaxis should be taken for the whole of this first trip, by when the situation will be known.

Antimalarial chemoprophylaxis is advised for those workers on oil rigs based in river estuaries.

Offshore rigs pose little risk and antimalarial chemoprophylaxis may only be needed if staying overnight onshore during transit.

7.6 Visits to national parks

Travellers visiting countries where malaria is restricted in distribution may plan to make day trips to national parks in malarious regions of the country. They should be advised on awareness of risk, bite precautions and the need for prompt attention in the event of fever during the succeeding year.
If they plan to stay overnight in the malarious area, e.g. in a safari lodge, they should also take chemoprophylaxis.

7.7 Stopovers

Many stopovers are in urban or tourist areas (particularly in Asia) and have minimal malaria risk. They are often situated in countries which may have malaria transmission in parts. Therefore, in order to assess risk it is essential to establish where overnight accommodation will be.

Stopovers in most of Sub-Saharan Africa, including main cities, present a risk of malaria and antimalarial prophylaxis should be recommended.

7.8 Last minute travellers

Last minute visits to malarious regions, whether for vacation, business or family reasons, are now commonplace.
This may leave the traveller little time to seek and act on travel advice.

Retail pharmacy outlets can supply over-the-counter antimalarials (chloroquine and/or proguanil) and antimosquito products, but mefloquine, doxycycline and atovaquone/proguanil are currently prescription only medicines (POMs).

If the traveller cannot obtain a GP appointment at short notice, some commercial travel clinics cater for walk-in attendees.

Doxycycline or atovaquone/proguanil should be started 2 days before travel to a malarious area. Chloroquine or proguanil or chloroquine plus proguanil one week before, and mefloquine 2-3 weeks before (to ensure tolerance). *Nevertheless, it is better to start chemoprophylaxis late than not to take it at all, as suppressive prophylactics will begin to work by the end of the incubation period.*

Where the recommended choice for the region to be visited is mefloquine or doxycycline or atovaquone/proguanil, it would be sensible to avoid mefloquine for last-minute prophylaxis if the traveller has not taken and tolerated mefloquine in the past.

ACMP does not recommend loading doses of any prophylactic antimalarial. The dosages recommended in these guidelines should be followed.

7.9 Visiting friends and relatives

(Adapted from the HPA Travel and Migrant Health Report 2006[67])

In the UK, malaria predominantly affects the non UK born population and their families, particularly those from Africa and south Asia, largely due to their high rates of travel to malarious areas.

Data suggest that people visiting friends and relatives are significantly less likely to take antimalarial prophylaxis than other travellers to Africa. Reasons for this may be that those visiting friends and relatives in Africa substantially underestimate the risk of acquiring malaria, and overestimate the amount of protection that having been brought up in Africa may give them.

Awareness needs to be raised that malaria is not a trivial disease. Those born in malarious countries need to be aware that any immunity they may have acquired is rapidly lost after migration to the UK. The view that this group is relatively protected is a dangerous myth. Migrants from malarious areas also need to be made aware that second-generation members of their families have no clinically relevant immunity of any kind to malaria, and that their children are particularly vulnerable.

Effective chemoprophylaxis taken correctly should reduce the risk of malaria by around 90%, especially if combined with sleeping under insecticide-treated nets.

Appropriately tailored health information should be targeted to migrant communities, especially of African descent, to stress the importance of chemoprophylaxis. Health advisers for this group, including primary care practitioners working in areas with large numbers of migrants, can have a major role to play.

Those who feel unwell following any trip to tropical areas should be encouraged to present to their doctors early, and to inform the doctors that they are at risk of malaria. Patients of African origin, and occasionally even doctors, can underestimate the severity of malaria in this group.

7.10 Students and children at boarding school

Many people from malaria-endemic areas come to the UK for secondary or higher education.

Those who stay in Britain for a year or more will lose a significant degree of any malarial immunity they had acquired and become more susceptible to clinical malaria. When they return home they should be advised as for the section on long term visitors to the UK returning to live in malarious parts of the world.

Those who are making short visits home (e.g. in school or college vacations) should be considered as VFR travellers and should be advised to use chemoprophylaxis in addition to personal protective measures against mosquito bites.

Students may become infected during their school or college vacations but the first symptoms of clinical malaria may actually occur in term time whilst they are in the UK. Therefore, it is essential that school/college nursing and medical staff consider malaria from the outset in any pupil from, or with a history of travel to, a malarious region and arrange a blood test for malaria without delay.

7.11 The long-term traveller

7.11.1 Risk assessment

The long term traveller is defined here as those travelling through, or visiting malaria-endemic countries for over six months.

One major problem for the long-term traveller is the variable access to and quality of medical care available overseas[68]. The provision of details of healthcare facilities or points of information could be crucial.

The main issues influencing the choice of malaria chemoprophylaxis on a long-term basis are the same as for short-term use, i.e. malaria risk, adverse events profile, compliance and efficacy. However, the licensing criteria for antimalarial drugs often restrict the recommended periods of administration (usually due to a lack of formal trials of long-term administration, rather than from evidence of adverse effects). This leads to uncertainly about the safety of long-term prescribing.

A decision on whether chemoprophylaxis is continued on a long-term basis may be influenced by the overall length of stay, seasonal risk in the area, and access to medical facilities. Travellers living or backpacking in rural areas may be far from appropriate medical attention and the need for standby emergency medication should also be considered. The continued use of chemoprophylaxis will also depend on current personal health, current medication, previous medical history, pregnancy, and relevant family medical history. However, long-term travellers are at high risk from malaria, and should not neglect necessary prophylaxis.

Health risks for the long-term traveller will vary considerably, depending in part on the reasons for travel including:

Visiting friends and relatives (VFR)

Individuals who originate from countries where malaria is transmitted, but who have settled in the UK. They may later visit their country of origin and remain there for long periods of time while working or visiting friends and relatives. They may perceive little risk from malaria infection or believe they are immune. This is not true (see section on VFR in this chapter).

Expatriates

Usually based at a single location where the risk of malaria is known, they often have access to medical care, a good standard of accommodation and are usually more aware of the malaria risks. However, up to 30% of some expatriates develop malaria within two years and many cases can be attributed to poor compliance with prophylaxis[69].

Backpackers

Often younger than expatriates, they may be less careful of their personal safety and less adherent to medical advice, in addition to having less experience of overseas travel in general. They have less control over their environment as they are constantly moving on.

7.11.2 Chemoprophylaxis for long-term travellers

Adverse events

The cumulative risk of contracting malaria is roughly proportional to the length of stay in a malarious area over the first few months. A three-month visit carries a risk around six times greater than a visit of two weeks.

Whilst the risk of new adverse events falls off over time, the risk of contracting malaria continues to increase roughly linearly as exposure to malaria continues (see figure 8). Thus, chemoprophylaxis in highly malarious areas is even more important for long-term visitors than it is for short-term travellers. Indeed, long-term travellers may wish to consider using malaria prophylaxis, or have standby medication, when short-term travellers might not, because of their sustained exposure to a small risk of infection.

Adherence to chemoprophylaxis

Compliance has been shown to decrease with the duration of travel[70], except where military-style discipline tends to support compliance. There is also evidence of weekly regimens having increased compliance over daily regimens[70].

Possible reasons for reduced compliance in long-term travellers may include:
- Fear of long-term side effects.
- Actual adverse events on one or more regimens.
- Conflicting advice.
- Complex regimen/daily tablets.
- Reduced confidence if intercurrent fever misdiagnosed as malaria.
- Perception from anecdotal evidence that chemoprophylaxis is unnecessary[71].

In addition, long-term travellers may overlook personal protective measures against mosquitoes[72].

FIGURE 8   CUMULATIVE RISK OF ADVERSE EVENTS AND OF MALARIA

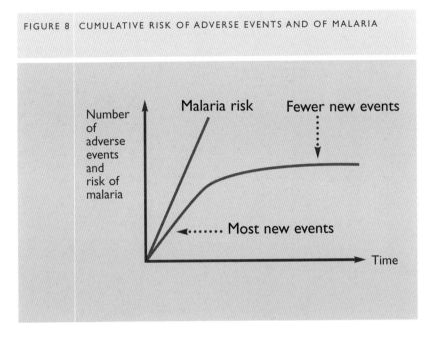

Efficacy of regimens

It is important to stress that no chemoprophylactic regimen is 100% effective and that anti-mosquito measures should also be used. Travellers should be encouraged to continue chemoprophylaxis despite suffering what they believe to be a malarial illness. Many febrile episodes in long-term travellers or expatriates are incorrectly diagnosed as malaria.

Licensing restrictions

The specific problem relating to prophylaxis advice for long-term travellers is that long-term use of many of the currently advised malaria drugs falls outside the terms of their current Marketing Authorisation (Licence).

There have been a number of approaches in response to this time limit:

- Switching from one chemoprophylactic regimen to another as the time limit is reached.

- Using chloroquine and proguanil, the only regimen licensed for long-term use but considered to give suboptimal protection in areas of markedly chloroquine-resistant falciparum malaria.

- Discontinuing prophylaxis in favour of access to local advice and standby or physician-guided treatment.

- Continuing with one prophylactic regimen beyond its licensed length of use.

General advice for all regimens

- Once an individual is compliant on one prophylactic regimen and is tolerating it well, transfer to another regimen increases the likelihood of the development of side effects due to the introduction of a different drug.
- There is no evidence of new side effects emerging during long-term use of any currently available prophylactics, though it is often thought that there may be risks associated with long-term use of chloroquine, see below.
- Evidence for safety in long-term use comes more from an accumulating lack of evidence of harm than from scientific evidence of safety.
- Individual risk assessments are important when deciding what advice should be given. In particular advice on prophylaxis may be influenced by other measures that might be used by those staying in areas where the risk is seasonally variable.
- Simplicity in regimen can, as always, be expected to improve compliance. The safest option is compliance with one of the most effective regimens.
- Minimising exposure to infection is important, especially taking precautions against being bitten whilst asleep.
- It is essential to seek medical advice promptly if symptoms develop.

ACMP advice on long-term use of specific antimalarials is summarised in table 16.

7.11.3 Specific considerations for women

See section on pregnancy and breastfeeding in chapter 6 which includes advice on chemprophylaxis prior to conception.

7.11.4 Specific considerations for infants and older children

Refer to section on children above.

Evidence in support of long-term use of antimalarials in infants and older children is limited. Advice for long-term use in these age groups is the same as for adults.

- Chloroquine: safe for both infants and young children.
- Proguanil: safe for use by infants and young children[73].
- Mefloquine: well tolerated[74]. Long-term use of mefloquine is reported to be safe, well tolerated and not associated with an increase in adverse effects[75-77].
- Doxycycline: Not for use in those under 12 years of age. No data available on the long-term use of doxycycline; however, long-term use of other tetracyclines for other indications is generally well tolerated[78].
- Atovaquone plus proguanil: both highly effective and safe[42].

7.12 Long term visitors to the UK returning to live in malarious parts of the world

Persons returning to their original homes in malarious regions after prolonged residence in the UK are likely to have suffered a decline in the partial immunity to malaria that develops during childhood and is maintained by repeated exposure in endemic regions. They may

TABLE 16   LONG TERM CHEMOPROPHYLAXIS FOR ADULTS UPDATED
FROM THE 2003 ACMP GUIDELINES ON MALARIA
PROPHYLAXIS FOR LONG-TERM TRAVELLERS[55]

MALARIA CHEMOPROPHYLAXIS	ACMP ADVICE ON LONG-TERM USE
Chloroquine	Considered safe for long-term use.* Consider ophthalmic examination 6 to 12 monthly, commencing at 6 years' prophylactic usage.
Proguanil	Considered safe for long-term use.*
Mefloquine	No evidence of harm in long-term use if tolerated in the short term. Suggest can be used safely for up to three years in the absence of side effects.
Doxycycline	No evidence of harm in long-term use. Evidence suggests that it may be used safely for periods of at least up to two years.
Atovaquone/ Proguanil	No evidence of harm in long-term use. Suggest can be used confidently for travel up to one year and possibly longer, but only with caution until more post-licensing experience is available.

* Considered safe for long-term use but considerable concern regarding level of
protective efficacy of the combination of chloroquine plus proguanil in certain
geographical areas where the regimen used to be useful

TABLE 17   HALF-LIVES OF SELECTED ANTIMALARIAL DRUGS

DRUG	HALF-LIFE
Chloroquine	Can extend from 6 to 60 days
Mefloquine	2 to 3 weeks
Doxycycline	12 to 24 hours
Atovaquone	2 to 3 days
Proguanil	14 to 21 hours

therefore be at increased risk of suffering an acute attack of malaria after returning home.

Pregnant women and small children are at higher risk than others of suffering severe disease.

Risk assessment and personal counselling is essential to warn individuals of the risk of suffering from malaria, emphasising avoidance measures, and the need for immediate diagnosis and treatment of acute feverish illnesses.

7.12.1 Preventive measures appropriate to an endemic setting[79]

Bed nets
Bed nets and other personal barrier protective measures (e.g. suitable clothing) are very low-cost, are effective long-term, have virtually no side-effects and will also help to protect from other mosquito-borne infections.

Intermittent Preventive Therapy (IPT)
If IPT is local policy in their destination country to prevent malaria in pregnancy and childhood, the returning visitor should be advised to seek medical advice on this immediately on arrival.

Case management of illness
People should be advised to seek medical attention immediately if either they or their children become feverish after repatriation in the endemic country. They should be warned that a malaria attack may be more serious because of diminished immunity.

Guidance
See the World Health Organization/ national country guidance on the appropriate measures in endemic settings which include IPT, insecticide-treated bednets and case-management of illness with therapy.

7.12.2 Prophylaxis

Intended use
The ACMP prophylaxis guidance is for temporary protection for the UK traveller. This is not appropriate for individuals who are returning to permanent residence in their country of origin.

Exception for pregnant women and young children
A limited period of prophylaxis of four to six weeks for pregnant women and young children may be appropriate in some circumstances, to allow them to settle and arrange for future healthcare after arrival in the endemic country.

Standby treatment
Offering standby treatment is inappropriate where there are likely to be health services to diagnose and manage malaria.

8 - Frequently Asked Questions

8.1
What malaria prevention should be advised for travellers going on cruises? — 85

8.2
What alternative antimalarial drugs can be used for India (and Sri Lanka) if chloroquine and proguanil are unsuitable for a traveller? — 85

8.3
Which antimalarial can I give to a traveller with a history of psoriasis? — 86

8.4
Which antimalarial can I give a traveller who is taking warfarin? — 86

8.5
How long is it safe to continue a course of antimalarial tablets? — 87

8.6
Which antimalarial drugs are suitable for women during pregnancy? — 88

8.7
Which antimalarial drugs can be taken by breastfeeding women? — 89

8.8
Which malaria drugs can be given to babies and young children? — 89

8.9
What is the easiest way to calculate the correct dose of chloroquine for babies and young children? — 90

8.10
Many travellers I see intend to travel through several areas where different anti-malarials are recommended as they progress through their journey. How do we advise these travellers? — 90

8.11
Which antimalarial drugs can I advise for a traveller who has epilepsy? — 91

8.12
What do I advise for the traveller with Glucose 6-phosphate dehydrogenase deficiency? — 91

8.13
What do I advise people working on oil rigs? — 92

8.14
What do I advise for the traveller on a stopover? — 92

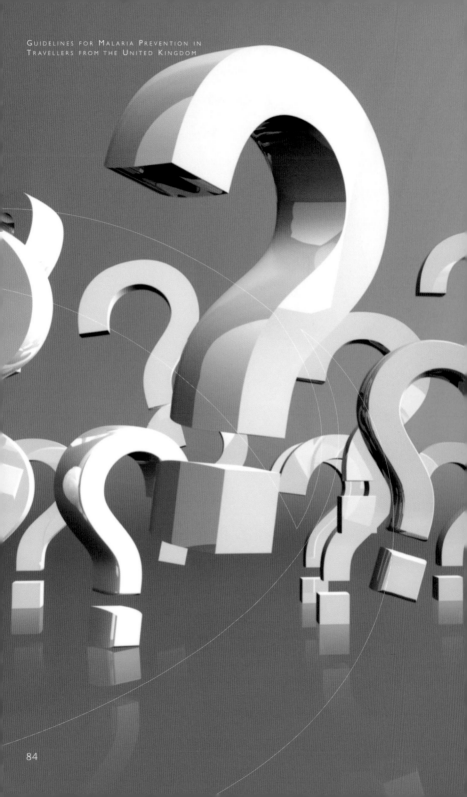

8. Frequently Asked Questions

Q1. What malaria prevention should be advised for travellers going on cruises?

A. Cruises are a growing part of the holiday market. Most travellers on cruises are only ashore during daylight hours when the *Anopheles* vector of malaria is not feeding, and therefore do not require malaria chemoprophylaxis. Occasionally this is not the case and therefore the cruise itinerary must be reviewed to determine if there will be exposure to malaria.

As examples, cruises in the Caribbean may include several days travelling along the Amazon in Brazil, or Orinoco River in Venezuela. Cruises along the East African coast may include a stop for a night or more in the port of Mombasa, Kenya and passengers may be ashore or on deck after dusk. These itineraries will require malaria chemoprophylaxis.

In addition cruises that have an overnight stay in any other malaria endemic region of the world require malaria chemoprophylaxis. Risks in specific destinations can be determined by referring to the country tables 7-12 in chapter 4.
Based on the destination, duration of exposure, and health of the traveller, the choice of malaria chemoprophylaxis can be made using the advice in these guidelines.
All travellers on cruises should use insect bite avoidance measures (see chapter 3).

Q2. What alternative antimalarial drugs can be used for India (and Sri Lanka) if chloroquine and proguanil are unsuitable for a traveller?

A. Chloroquine plus proguanil are the recommended chemoprophylaxis for India (apart from Assam state in Northern India where either mefloquine, doxycycline or atovaquone/proguanil are the drugs of choice) and Sri Lanka. If a traveller is unable to take the combination of chloroquine plus proguanil, the alternative is a choice between one of three prescription drugs available: mefloquine, doxycycline or atovaquone/proguanil.

It depends on the reason why chloroquine and proguanil are not suitable as to which alternative is considered (e.g. those unable to take chloroquine due to epilepsy should not take mefloquine; if a traveller does not tolerate proguanil, then they should avoid atovaqone/proguanil (Malarone®) as this also contains proguanil). For advice on malaria prevention in pregnant women there is a specific FAQ below.

Chloroquine plus proguanil remain the first choice agents in India and Sri Lanka because for most areas in these countries, *Plasmodium vivax* is the most prevalent species of malaria present and chloroquine is highly effective against this species. Because there is some *P. falciparum* present, the addition of proguanil to chloroquine provides additional protection against strains of *P. falciparum* that may be resistant to chloroquine alone. Where there is frequent or high level resistance, such as the Assam region discussed above, alternative agents are used.

85

Q3. Which antimalarial can I give to a traveller with a history of psoriasis?

A. Proguanil, atovaquone/proguanil, doxycycline and mefloquine do not cause problems in those with psoriasis. Chloroquine and chloroquine-related drugs can exacerbate psoriasis and should be avoided in those with generalised psoriasis or a history of such. Travellers with mild psoriasis can consider chloroquine if they are aware of the possible risks. The benefit of chemoprophylaxis with chloroquine may outweigh the risk of exacerbation of psoriasis, but each case should be considered on an individual basis.

Q4. Which antimalarial can I give a traveller who is taking warfarin?

A. Travellers on anticoagulants should ensure their clotting time is stable prior to departure. It should be noted that patients on warfarin may have underlying cardiac disease and may be on cardiac medication. Interactions with other medication together with the individuals' medical history should be taken into account when deciding on appropriate malaria chemoprophylaxis.

Documented interactions between warfarin and antimalarial tablets

Chloroquine

There is no interaction between warfarin and chloroquine documented in the BNF, although there is a caution in the Summary of Product Characteristics for Nivaquine.

Proguanil

There has been an isolated report of an enhanced effect of warfarin when taken together with proguanil[58].

Mefloquine

Mefloquine is not considered to be a problem for those taking warfarin. The manufacturer states that '*although no drug interaction is known with anticoagulants, effects of mefloquine on travellers should be checked before departure.*'
Please see below for how this can be monitored.

Atovaquone/proguanil (Malarone®)

It is unknown whether there are interactions between Malarone and warfarin, although there have been isolated reports of an enhanced effect of warfarin when taken together with proguanil (see above under proguanil).

Doxycycline

The anticoagulant effect of coumarins (including warfarin) is possibly enhanced by tetracyclines[59].

Advice for travellers needing malaria chemoprophylaxis who are taking warfarin

Travellers should start taking their malaria tablets at least 1 week (and ideally 2-3 weeks in the case of mefloquine) prior to their departure. A baseline INR should be checked prior to starting chemoprophylaxis, and re-checked after 1 week of taking chemoprophylaxis. If a traveller is away for a long period of time the INR should be checked at intervals at the destination. However, the sensitivity of thromboplastin reagent used by some laboratories in different countries may vary[60].

Q5. How long can a traveller take different antimalarial drugs?

A. Guidelines for the long term use of malaria tablets are summarised in chapter 7 and were originally published in 2003 by the ACMP[55].

The main issues influencing the choice of malaria chemoprophylaxis on a long-term basis are the same as for short-term, i.e. adverse event profile, ease of compliance and efficacy. However, the specific issue relating to advice on chemoprophylaxis for the long-term traveller relates to current licensing restrictions. Long term use of malaria chemoprophylaxis outside licensing restrictions is based on the cumulative evidence of lack of harm rather than positive evidence of safety. This situation is unlikely to change.

Chloroquine
Chloroquine has been taken safely for periods of many years at doses used for malaria chemoprophylaxis. However, there has been concern expressed about the possible development of retinal toxicity with long term use of chloroquine (or hydroxychloroquine, often used to treat rheumatologic disorders). Retinal toxicity has been described in those on daily chloroquine dosage for rheumatic disorders. As a result, two thresholds for the risk of retinopathy have been suggested:
* A total cumulative dose of 100g of chloroquine base
* A daily dose of 250mg base (4mg/kg)[80].

The first threshold would require an adult to take chloroquine continuously, weekly, for a period of six years. The second threshold is far in excess of the prophylactic dosage. It has been concluded that the risk of retinopathy from prophylactic dosage alone is negligible[29]. Further reassurance can be gained from the fact that retinopathy has only rarely been reported in patients taking weekly prophylactic dosages[80,81].

ACMP advice suggests that chloroquine can be taken on a long-term basis. However, physicians should consider an ophthalmologic examination every 6 -12 months , beginning at 6 years' cumulative use for those on long-term chloroquine.

Proguanil
There is no time limit specified for the use of proguanil. Therefore, it can be taken continuously for several years.

Mefloquine
There are few data on the use of mefloquine for periods exceeding two years, although there is no evidence of cumulative toxicity, and mefloquine taken for over 1 year is well tolerated. The product licence suggests mefloquine can be taken continuously for a period of up to 12 months. However, advice from the ACMP indicates that there is no evidence of harm in long term use if the drug is tolerated in the short term, and suggests that mefloquine can be used safely for up to three years in the absence of side effects.

Doxycycline
Doxycycline is licensed for up to two years or more in the treatment of acne in the same dose as is used for malaria prophylaxis. The ACMP have concluded that there is no evidence of harm in long-term use of doxycycline and it may be taken safely for periods of at least up to two years.

Atovaquone/proguanil (Malarone®)
Both components of Malarone® have been used individually on a long term basis, although there is little experience of long-term use of the combination. Many countries do not restrict the length of time atovaquone/proguanil can be taken although the UK product license states it can only be taken for travel up to 28 days.

There is a report of atovaquone/proguanil use for periods from 9 to 34 weeks, in which there was no excess of adverse effects and no appearance of unexpected adverse effects[82]. The ACMP concludes that there is no evidence of harm in long-term use and suggests that it can be taken confidently for travel up to one year or longer. Nevertheless, long-term use of atovaquone/proguanil should be prescribed with careful consideration until additional post licensing experience is available.

Q6. Which antimalarial drugs are suitable for women during pregnancy?

A. Malaria during pregnancy is a serious illness for both the mother and the fetus. Pregnant women should be advised against travel to an area with malaria, particularly it there is chloroquine resistant *Plasmodium falciparum*.

Doxycycline and atovaquone/proguanil (Malarone®) are both unsuitable for use during pregnancy.

Results of animal studies indicate that tetracyclines cross the placenta, are found in fetal tissues and can have toxic effects on the developing foetus (often related to retardation of skeletal development). Evidence of embryotoxicity has also been noted in animals treated early in pregnancy (SPC).

The safety of atovaquone and proguanil hydrochloride when administered concurrently for use in human pregnancy has not been established and the potential risk is unknown. Animal studies showed no evidence for teratogenicity of the combination. The individual components have shown no adverse effects on parturition or pre- and post-natal development (SPC). Women should be reassured that taking Malarone inadvertently prior to or during the first trimester is not an indication to terminate a pregnancy.

The data available from studies on the prophylactic use of mefloquine in pregnancy is generally reassuring. Most experts recommend that mefloquine is avoided during the first trimester, but can be offered to women during the second and third trimesters. The risk of adverse effects of mefloquine use in pregnancy should be balanced against the risk of contracting malaria and the complications that can result.
The decision on whether to recommend mefloquine should be carefully discussed with the traveller.

Women of childbearing age should take contraceptive precautions while taking mefloquine and for three months after the last dose. However, they should be reassured that taking mefloquine inadvertently prior to or during the first trimester is not an indication to terminate a pregnancy.

Both chloroquine and proguanil have been taken safely during pregnancy for many years although this combination offers insufficient protection in areas with chloroquine resistant *P. falciparum*. Folic acid supplements should be taken if proguanil is used in those who are pregnant or seeking to become pregnant.

Q7. Which antimalarial drugs can be taken by breastfeeding women?

A. Breastfeeding women should not take doxycycline or atovaquone/proguanil (Malarone®). Chloroquine plus proguanil can be used during breastfeeding although this combination provides suboptimal protection for the mother in areas of chloroquine resistant *Plasmodium falciparum* malaria.

There is little data on the use of mefloquine during breastfeeding (see Breastfeeding section in chapter 6). Although mefloquine is excreted in breast milk in small amounts there is not enough data to draw conclusions regarding potential harmful effects on the infant.

Mefloquine may be considered for breastfeeding mothers travelling to areas of chloroquine resistant *P. falciparum*. Each traveller should be assessed individually, weighing the potential risks and benefits of taking mefloquine whilst breastfeeding, and taking into consideration the risk of malaria at the destination.

The small amounts of antimalarials that pass into breast milk are not enough to protect the baby. Breastfeeding infants therefore need to take their own prophylaxis. If both mother and infant are taking mefloquine there is a concern that the amount of mefloquine the infant may receive will exceed the recommended maximum, particularly in infants in the lower weight range. However, this possible effect is likely to be short lasting as the weight of the child increases and the contribution of mefloquine in breast milk to the total prophylactic dose becomes relatively small.

Q8. Which antimalarial drugs can be given to babies and young children?

A. Both chloroquine and proguanil can be given from birth. Chloroquine is available as syrup but proguanil will need to be crushed and given with jam or food.

Mefloquine can be given to infants weighing 5 kg or more (see Summary of Product Characteristics). Atovaquone/proguanil (Malarone®) can be given to infants weighing 11 kg or more; paediatric tablets are available.

Doxycycline is unsuitable for children under 12 years.

One of the main challenges in giving malaria tablets to babies and young children will be the practical aspects of administration.

All dosages for malaria chemoprophylaxis in children are found in tables 4-6 in chapter 4 and in the British National Formulary (BNF). The dose for children will be dependent on the weight/age of the infant or child.

Mosquito bite avoidance is extremely important for this age group.

Q9. What is the easiest way to calculate the correct dose of chloroquine for babies and young children?

A. The dose steps for chloroquine syrup are not the same as for chloroquine tablets and a child may be prescribed a different dose of chloroquine depending on whether they take tablets or syrup (see tables 4 and 5, chapter 4). The main reason for any differences is due to the different amount of chloroquine base within the syrup and the tablets. The chloroquine syrup formulation contains 50 mg chloroquine base/5 mls syrup. The amount of chloroquine base contained within the tablets is 150mg (Nivaquine) and 155mg (Avloclor).

An additional factor which might be confusing is that the packet insert for chloroquine phosphate (Avloclor) gives different dosages (usually lower) for children than in these guidelines and the BNF. The ACMP guidelines and BNF dosages should be used.

While there is an optimum dose of chloroquine base for children of every weight, the final dosage given to the child will depend, in part, on the practicality of administering the formulation of chloroquine available (i.e. either tablet or syrup). E.g., when dividing tablets for children, it is not possible to break a tablet into thirds, so the dosages will involve either a half or a quarter of a tablet.

The tables in chapter 4 have been calculated based on weight and surface area and the most accurate dose according to the weight is recommended. Although differences occur, all recommended dosages in the tables fall within accepted limits of toxicity. It is important not to overdose children with chloroquine as severe toxicity can occur.

A practical approach when calculating children's dosages for chloroquine is to decide on the most appropriate preparation (either tablet or syrup) for the child and calculate the dose appropriate to that preparation, according to the tables in chapter 4.

Q10. Many travellers I see are travelling through areas where different anti-malarials are recommended as they progress through their journey. How do we advise these travellers?

A. Travellers planning extensive journeys across continents will often travel into areas which have different malaria chemoprophylaxis recommendations. In these situations it is important that the traveller is protected in all areas of risk and the choice of medication needs to reflect the overall risk.

It may be possible to move from one regimen to another, although for shorter trips this may not be practical. For example, a traveller visiting parts of India for 2 weeks (where chloroquine plus proguanil may be recommended) and then going on to areas in Myanmar and Cambodia for 6 weeks (where mefloquine, doxycycline or atovaquone/proguanil may be recommended) would be advised to take either mefloquine, doxycycline or atovaquone/proguanil for the whole of the visit rather than change from chloroquine and proguanil to one of the other agents.

Q11. Which antimalarial drugs can I advise for a traveller who has epilepsy?

A. Both chloroquine and mefloquine are unsuitable for those with epilepsy. For areas with a high risk of chloroquine resistant *Plasmodium falciparum*, doxycycline or atovaquone/proguanil can be used. However for children under the age of 12 the only suitable antimalarials under these circumstances will be atovaquone/proguanil (Malarone®) (bearing in mind the length of travel). Proguanil alone can be given for malarious areas without chloroquine resistance.

Phenytoin, carbamazepine and barbiturates reduce the half life of doxycycline; in theory the dose should be increased for those taking these drugs. However, there is no evidence that this is necessary, and a dose adjustment is not recommended.

Q12. What do I advise for the traveller with Glucose 6-phosphate dehydrogenase deficiency?

A. Glucose 6-phosphate dehydrogenase (G6PD) is an enzyme in the hexose monophosphate shunt of the glycolytic pathway. This shunt supports the red cell's protection against oxidative damage. Absence of G6PD renders the red cell liable to haemolysis in the presence of some drugs.

The most common G6PD deficiency allele in Africa (G6PD A-) has been shown to confer some resistance to malaria in both hemizygous males and heterozygous females[61]. Nevertheless, all G6PD-deficient travellers to malarious areas still require appropriate chemoprophylaxis.

Chloroquine
There is a theoretical risk of haemolysis in some G6PD-deficient individuals who receive chloroquine. This risk is acceptable in acute malaria[59] and G6PD levels are not usually checked before using chloroquine in treatment doses. Haemolysis does not appear to be a problem when chloroquine is given in the dose recommended for malaria chemoprophylaxis so there is no need to withhold chloroquine prophylaxis from those known to be G6PD-deficient.

Primaquine
This drug is not currently recommended as a first line agent for malaria prevention in UK travellers, but may be considered in special circumstances on expert advice[27]. There is a definite risk of haemolysis in G6PD-deficient individuals. The traveller's G6PD level must be checked before primaquine is prescribed and G6PD deficiency contraindicates its use for prophylaxis.

Q13. What do I advise people working on oil rigs?

A. There is a large number of staff employed in the oil industry predominantly based around West Africa. Employees commonly travel to these areas every 4-6 weeks, followed by a similar period of leave back in the UK. Oil rigs may be based in river estuaries or many miles offshore. Therefore the level of risk may be difficult to assess until one period of work has been completed and antimalarial chemoprophylaxis should be taken for the whole of this first trip.

Antimalarial chemoprophylaxis is advised for those workers on oil rigs based in river estuaries.

Offshore rigs pose little risk and antimalarial chemoprophylaxis may only be needed if staying overnight onshore during transit.

Q14. What do I advise for the traveller on a stopover?

A. Many stopovers are in urban or tourist areas (particularly in Asia) and have minimal malaria risk. They are often situated in countries which may have malaria transmission in parts. Therefore, in order to assess risk it is essential to establish where overnight accommodation will be.

Stopovers in most of sub-Saharan Africa, including main cities, present a risk of malaria and antimalarial prophylaxis should be recommended.

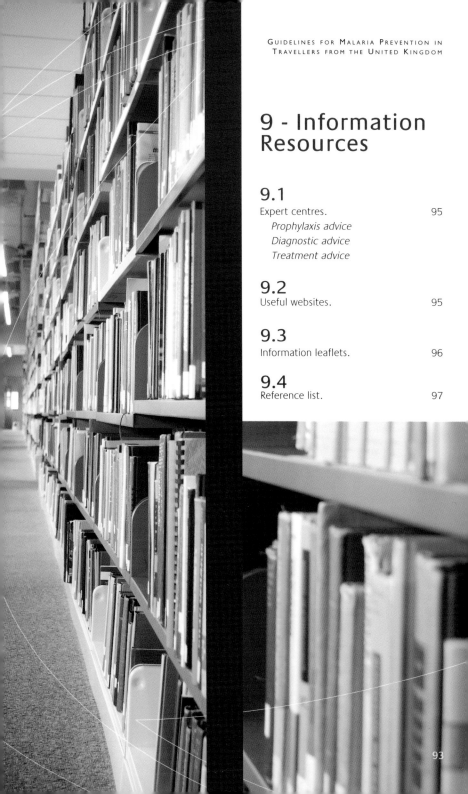

9 - Information Resources

9.1
Expert centres.   95
  Prophylaxis advice
  Diagnostic advice
  Treatment advice

9.2
Useful websites.   95

9.3
Information leaflets.   96

9.4
Reference list.   97

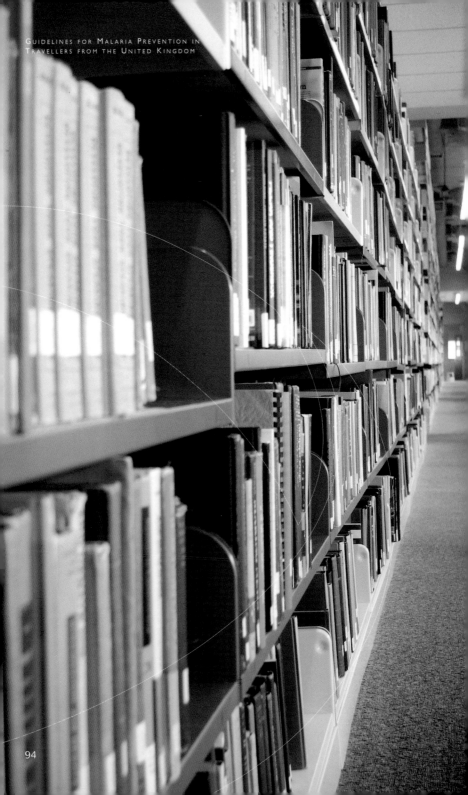

9. Information Resources

9.1 Expert centres

9.1.1 Prophylaxis advice

Malaria Reference Laboratory (MRL)
http://www.malaria-reference.co.uk
Advice line for healthcare professionals:
020 7636 3924

National Travel Health Network and Centre
(NaTHNaC)   http://www.nathnac.org/
Advice line for healthcare professionals:
0845 602 6712

Liverpool School of Tropical Medicine (LSTM)
http://www.liv.ac.uk/lstm/

TRAVAX (Health Protection Scotland)
http://www.travax.nhs.uk/

9.1.2 Diagnostic advice

Malaria Reference Laboratory (MRL)
http://www.malaria-reference.co.uk
Diagnostic advice for health care professionals
020 7927 2427

The Hospital for Tropical Diseases (HTD)
http://www.thehtd.org/

The Liverpool School of Tropical Medicine
(LSTM)   http://www.liv.ac.uk/lstm/
Advice line for Healthcare professionals
0151 708 9393

9.1.3 Treatment advice

The treatment of malaria is outside the scope
of this document and will be addressed in
ACMP malaria treatment guidelines.
Expert advice on malaria treatment may be
obtained from:

The Hospital for Tropical Diseases (HTD)
http://www.thehtd.org/
Requests for emergency admission or very
urgent clinic attendance should be made to
the Duty Doctor, who is bleeped via
switchboard. Telephone: 0845 1555 000
Bleep 5845

The Liverpool School of Tropical Medicine
(LSTM)   http://www.liv.ac.uk/lstm/
Advice line for Healthcare professionals
0151 708 9393

Your local infectious diseases unit

British Infection Society (BIS)
http://www.britishinfectionsociety.org/
(malaria treatment algorithm)

9.2 Useful websites

British National Formulary (BNF)
http://www.bnf.org

British Infection Society (BIS)
http://www.britishinfectionsociety.org/

Department of Health
http://www.dh.gov.uk

Electronic Medicines Compendium
(for Summaries of Product Characteristics)
http://www.emc.medicines.org

Liverpool School of Tropical Medicine (LSTM)
http://www.liv.ac.uk/lstm/

London School of Hygiene and Tropical
Medicine (LSHTM)
http://www.lshtm.ac.uk/

Malaria Reference Laboratory (MRL)
http://www.malaria-reference.co.uk

Medicines and Healthcare products Regulatory
Agency (MHRA)
http://www.mhra.gov.uk

National Travel Health Network and Centre
(NaTHNaC)
http://www.nathnac.org/

Health Protection Agency (HPA)
http://www.hpa.org.uk/

Royal Society of Tropical Medicine and
Hygiene (RSTM&H)
http://www.rstmh.org/

TRAVAX (Health Protection Scotland)
http://www.travax.nhs.uk/

World Health Organization (WHO)
International Travel and Health
http://www.who.int/ith/en/

9.3 Information Leaflets

The Department of Health produces
"*Think Malaria*" leaflets, order code
MAL/1, which are available in 11 different
languages and can be obtained from the
DH Publications Orderline by writing to
DH Publications Orderline, PO Box 777
London SE1 6XH or telephoning 0870
155 5455 or by email to
dh@prolog.uk.com.

For further information please see the
Department of Health website
http://www.dh.gov.uk

9.4 References

1 General Medical Council. Good Medical Practice. General Medical Council, London 2001.

2 World Health Organization. World Malaria Report 2005. Geneva 2005.

3 White NJ. Manson's Tropical Diseases. Cook GC & Zumla A. (eds.), pp. 1242-8 Elsevier Science 2003.

4 Hay SI, Guerra CA, Tatem AJ, Atkinson PM, Snow RW. Urbanization, malaria transmission and disease burden in Africa. Nat Rev Microbiol. 2005;3:81-90.

5 Sharma VP. Current scenario of malaria in India. Parassitologia. 1999;41:349-53.

6 Maguire JD, Sumawinata IW, Masbar S et al. Chloroquine-resistant Plasmodium malariae in south Sumatra, Indonesia. Lancet. 2002;360:58-60.

7 Montemarano AD, Gupta RK, Burge JR, Klein K. Insect repellents and the efficacy of sunscreens. Lancet. 1997;349: 1670-1.

8 Murphy ME, Montemarano AD, Debboun M, Gupta R. The effect of sunscreen on the efficacy of insect repellent: a clinical trial. Journal American of the Academy of Dermatology. 2000;43:219-22.

9 McGready R, Hamilton KA, Simpson JA et al. Safety of the insect repellent N,N-diethyl-M-toluamide (DEET) in pregnancy. American Journal of Tropical Medicine & Hygiene. 2001;65:285-9.

10 Govere J, Durrheim DN, Baker L, Hunt R, Coetzee M. Efficacy of three insect repellents against the malaria vector Anopheles arabiensis. Medical & Veterinary Entomology. 2000;14:441-4.

11 Canadian recommendations for the prevention and treatment of malaria among international travellers. Canadian Communicable Disease Report. 2004;30 (Suppl 1):1-62.

12 Badolo A, Ilboudo-Sanogo E, Ouedraogo AP, Costantini C. Evaluation of the sensitivity of Aedes aegypti and Anopheles gambiae complex mosquitoes to two insect repellents: DEET and KBR 3023. Tropical Medicine International Health. 2004;9:330-4.

13 Costantini C, Badolo A, Ilboudo-Sanogo E. Field evaluation of the efficacy and persistence of insect repellents DEET, IR3535, and KBR 3023 against Anopheles gambiae complex and other Afrotropical vector mosquitoes. Transactions of the Royal Society of Tropical Medicine & Hygiene. 2004;98:644-52.

14 World Health Organization. Report of the fourth WHOPES working group meeting. WHO/CDS/WHOPES/2001.2. 2001. Geneva, World Health Organization.

15 No authors listed. Picardin - a new insect repellent. Medical Letters Drugs Therapy. 2005;47:46-7.

16 Fradin MS, Day JF. Comparative efficacy of insect repellents against mosquito bites. New England Journal Medicine. 2002;347:13-18.

17 Petersen E. Malaria chemoprophylaxis: when should we use it and what are the options? Expert Review Anti-Infective Therapy. 2004;2:119-32.

18 Lines JD, Myamba J, Curtis C F. Experimental hut trials of permethrin-impregnated mosquito nets and eave curtains against malaria vectors in Tanzania. Medical & Veterinary Entomology. 1987;1:37-51.

19 Schreck CE, Carlson DA, Weidhass DE. Wear and ageing tests with permethrin treated cotton polyester fabric. Journal of Economic Entomology. 1980;73:541-3.

20 Hewitt SE, Farham M, Urhaman H, Muhammed N, Kamal M, Rowland MW. Self-protection from malaria vectors in Pakistan: an evaluation of popular existing methods and appropriate new techniques in Afghan refugee communities. Annual Tropical Medicine & Parasitology. 1996; 90:337-44.

21 Khan AA, Maibach HI, Strauss WG, Fenley WR. Vitamin B1 is not a systemic mosquito repellent in man. Transactions of the St. Johns Hospital Dermatological Society. 1969;55:99-102.

22 Ives AR, Paskewitz SM. Testing vitamin B as a home remedy against mosquitoes. Journal of the American Mosquito Control Association. 2005;21:213-7.

23 Rajan TV, Hein M, Porte P, Wikel S. A double-blinded, placebo-controlled trial of garlic as a mosquito repellant: a preliminary study. Medical & Veterinary Entomology. 2005;19:84-9.

24 Dondorp AM, Newton PN, Mayxay M et al. Fake antimalarials in Southeast Asia are a major impediment to malaria control: multinational cross-sectional survey on the prevalence of fake antimalarials. Tropical Medicine International Health. 2004;9:1241-6.

25 Chulay JD. Challenges in the development of antimalarial drugs with causal prophylactic activity. Transactions of the Royal Society Of Tropical Medicine & Hygiene. 1998;92:577-9.

26 Franco-Paredes C, Santos-Preciado JI. Problem pathogens: prevention of malaria in travellers. Lancet Infectious Disease. 2006; 6:139-49.

27 Hill DR, Baird JK, Parise ME, Lewis LS, Ryan ET, Magill AJ. Primaquine: report from CDC expert meeting on malaria chemoprophylaxis I. American Journal of Tropical Medicine & Hygiene. 2006;75:402-15.

28 Pappaioanou M, Fishbein DB, Dreesen DW et al. Antibody response to preexposure human diploid-cell rabies vaccine given concurrently with chloroquine. New England Journal of Medicine. 1986;314:280-4.

29 Hill DR. Travel Associated Disease.
Cook GC (ed.), p. 101 Royal College
of Physicians, London,1995.

30 Limsomwong N, Pang LW, Singharaj P.
Malaria prophylaxis with proguanil in
children living in a malaria-endemic
area. American Journal of Tropical
Medicine & Hygiene. 1988;38:231-6.

31 Moore DA, Grant AD, Armstrong M,
Stumpfle R, Behrens RH. Risk factors
for malaria in UK travellers.
Transactions of the Royal Society of
Tropical Medicine & Hygiene.
2004;98:55-63.

32 Wongsrichanalai C, Pickard AL,
Wernsdorfer WH, Meshnick SR.
Epidemiology of drug-resistant
malaria. Lancet Infectious Diseases.
2002;2:209-18.

33 Schlagenhauf P, Tschopp A, Johnson R
et al. Tolerability of malaria
chemoprophylaxis in non-immune
travellers to sub-Saharan Africa:
multicentre, randomised, double
blind, four arm study. British Medical
Journal. 2003;327:1078.

34 Meier CR, Wilcock K, Jick SS. The risk
of severe depression, psychosis or
panic attacks with prophylactic
antimalarials. Drug Safety.
2004;27:203-13.

35 Wells TS, Smith TC, Smith B et al.
Mefloquine use and hospitalizations
among US service members, 2002-
2004. American Journal of Tropical
Medicine & Hygiene. 2006;74:744-9.

36 Taylor WR, White NJ. Antimalarial
drug toxicity: a review. Drug Safety.
2004;27, 25-61.

37 Ohrt, C, Richie TL, Widjaja H et al.
Mefloquine compared with
doxycycline for the prophylaxis of
malaria in Indonesian soldiers.
A randomized, double-blind,
placebo-controlled trial. Annals of
Internal Medicine. 1997;126:963-72.

38 Bryant SG, Fisher S, Kluge RM.
Increased frequency of doxycycline
side effects. Pharmacotherapy.
1987;7:125-9.

39 Edstein MD, Yeo AE, Kyle DE,
Looareesuwan S, Wilairatana P,
Rieckmann KH. Proguanil
polymorphism does not affect the
antimalarial activity of proguanil
combined with atovaquone in vitro.
Transactions of the Royal Society of
Tropical Medicine & Hygiene.
1996;90:418-21.

40 Berman JD, Nielsen R, Chulay JD.
Causal prophylactic efficacy of
atovaquone-proguanil (Malarone)
in a human challenge model.
Transactions of the Royal Society
of Tropical Medicine & Hygiene.
2001;95:429-32.

41 Camus D, Djossou F, Schilthuis HJ et al.
Atovaquone-proguanil versus
chloroquine-proguanil for malaria
prophylaxis in nonimmune pediatric
travelers: results of an international,
randomized, open-label study.
Clinical Infectious Diseases.
2004;38:1716-23.

42 Faucher JF, Binder R, Missinou MA et al.
Efficacy of atovaquone/proguanil for
malaria prophylaxis in children and its
effect on the immunogenicity of live
oral typhoid and cholera vaccines.
Clinical Infectious Diseases.
2002;35:1147-54.

43 Lell B, Luckner D, Ndjave M, Scott T, Kremsner PG. Randomised placebo-controlled study of atovaquone plus proguanil for malaria prophylaxis in children. Lancet. 1998;351:709-13.

44 Ling J, Baird JK, Fryauff DJ et al. Randomized, placebo-controlled trial of atovaquone/proguanil for the prevention of Plasmodium falciparum or Plasmodium vivax malaria among migrants to Papua, Indonesia. Clinical Infectious Diseases. 2002;35:825-33.

45 Marra F, Salzman JR, Ensom MH. Atovaquone-proguanil for prophylaxis and treatment of malaria. Annals of Pharmacotherapy. 2003;37:1266-75.

46 Overbosch D, Schilthuis H, Bienzle U et al. Atovaquone-proguanil versus mefloquine for malaria prophylaxis in nonimmune travelers: results from a randomized, double-blind study. Clinical Infectious Diseases. 2001;33:1015-21.

47 Shanks GD, Gordon DM, Klotz FW et al. Efficacy and safety of atovaquone/proguanil as suppressive prophylaxis for Plasmodium falciparum malaria. Clinical Infectious Diseases. 1998;27:494-9.

48 Sukwa TY, Mulenga M, Chisdaka N, Roskell NS, Scott TR. A randomized, double-blind, placebo-controlled field trial to determine the efficacy and safety of Malarone (atovaquone/proguanil) for the prophylaxis of malaria in Zambia. American Journal of Tropical Medicine & Hygiene. 1999;60:521-5.

49 Soto J, Toledo J, Luzz M, Gutierrez P, Berman J, Duparc S. Randomized, double-blind, placebo-controlled study of Malarone for malaria prophylaxis in non-immune Colombian soldiers. American Journal of Tropical Medicine & Hygiene. 2006;75:430-3.

50 Chen LH, Keystone JS. New strategies for the prevention of malaria in travelers. Infectious Disease Clinics of North America. 2005;19:185-210.

51 World Health Organization International travel and health. World Health Organization, Geneva, 2005.

52 Touze JE, Heno P, Fourcade L et al. The effects of antimalarial drugs on ventricular repolarization. American Journal of Tropical Medicine & Hygiene. 2002;67:54-60.

53 World Health Organization. The use of malaria rapid diagnostic tests. 2004. World Health Organization.

54 Jelinek T, Grobusch MP, Nothdurft HD. Use of dipstick tests for the rapid diagnosis of malaria in non-immune travelers. Journal of Travel Medicine. 2000;7:175-9.

55 Hughes C, Tucker R, Bannister B, Bradley DJ. Malaria prophylaxis for long-term travellers. Communicable Disease & Public Health. 2003;6:200-208.

56 Steketee RW, Wirima JJ, Slutsker L, Khoromana CO, Heymann DL, Breman JG. Malaria treatment and prevention in pregnancy: indications for use and adverse events associated with use of chloroquine or mefloquine. American Journal of Tropical Medicine & Hygiene. 1996;55(1 Suppl):50-56.

57 Nosten F, Vincenti M, Simpson J, Yei P, Thwai KL, de Vries A, Chongsuphajaisiddhi T, White NJ. The effects of mefloquine treatment in pregnancy. Clinical Infectious Diseases. 1999;28:808-15.

58 Armstrong G, Beg MF, Scahill S. Warfarin potentiated by proguanil. British Medical Journal.1991;303:789.

59 Joint Formulary Committee British National Formulary. British Medical Association and Royal Pharmaceutical Society of Great Britain. London, 2006.

60 Leon MN, Lateef M, Fuentes F. Prevention and Management of Cardiovascular Events during Travel. Journal of Travel Medicine. 1996;3:227-30.

61 Saunders MA, Hammer MF, Nachman MW. Nucleotide variability at G6PD and the signature of malarial selection in humans. Genetics. 2002;162:1849-61.

62 Serjeant GR. Infections in Sickle Cell Disease. In Cohen, J. & Powderly, WG (eds.) Infectious Diseases. p.1618. Mosby, Edinburgh, 2004.

63 Kotton CN, Ryan ET, Fishman JA. Prevention of infection in adult travelers after solid organ transplantation. American Journal of Transplantation. 2005;5:8-14.

64 Kamya MR, Gasasira AF, Yeka A et al. Effect of HIV-1 infection on antimalarial treatment outcomes in Uganda: a population-based study. Journal of Infectious Diseases. 2006;193:9-15.

65 Korenromp EL, Williams BG, de Vlas SJ et al. Malaria attributable to the HIV-1 epidemic, sub-Saharan Africa. Emerging Infectious Diseases. 2005;11:1410-19.

66 World Health Organization. Standards for maternal and neonatal care. 2004. World Health Organisation.

67 Health Protection Agency. Migrant Health: Infectious diseases in non-UK born populations in England, Wales and Northern Ireland. A baseline report – 2006. London: Health Protection Agency Centre for Infections. 2006.

68 Stenbeck JL. Health hazards in Swedish field personnel in the tropics. Travel Medicine International. 1991;9:51-9. 68. 69. Schneider I, Bradley DJ. 2003. Unpublished work.

70 Steffen R, Heusser R, Machler R et al. Malaria chemoprophylaxis among European tourists in tropical Africa: use, adverse reactions, and efficacy. Bulletin of the World Health Organization. 1990;68:313-22.

71 Janosi M. Advice to long-term travellers. Travel Medicine International. 1998;6:110-12.

72 Lobel HO, Phillips-Howard PA, Brandling-Bennett AD *et al*. Malaria incidence and prevention among European and north American travellers to Kenya. Bulletin of the World Health Organization. 1990;68:209-15.

73 Bruce-Chwatt LJ, Bruce-Chwatt JM. Antimalarial drugs in West Africa, with particular reference to proguanil; results of a survey in Nigeria. British Medical Journal. 1950;2:7-14.

74 Luxemburger C, Price RN, Nosten F, Ter Kuile FO, Chongsuphajaisiddhi T, White NJ. Mefloquine in infants and young children. Annals of Tropical Paediatrics. 1996;16:281-286.

75 Hopperus Buma AP, van Thiel PP, Lobel HO *et al*. Long-term malaria chemoprophylaxis with mefloquine in Dutch marines in Cambodia. Journal of Infectious Diseases. 1996;173:1506-9.

76 Lobel HO, Miani M, Eng T, Bernard KW, Hightower AW, Campbell CC. Long-term malaria prophylaxis with weekly mefloquine. Lancet. 1993;341:848-51.

77 Peragallo MS, Sabatinelli G, Sarnicola G. Compliance and tolerability of mefloquine and chloroquine plus proguanil for long-term malaria chemoprophylaxis in groups at particular risk (the military). Transactions of the Royal Society of Tropical Medicine & Hygiene. 1999;93:73-7.

78 Delaney TJ, Leppard BJ, MacDonald DM. Effects of long term treatment with tetracycline. Acta dermatovenereologica. 1974;54:487-9.

79 World Health Organization Factsheet No. 94 Malaria http://www.rbm.who.int/cmc_upload/0/000/015/369/RBMInfosheet_4.htm (accessed 15 Nov 2006)

80 Luzzi GA, Peto TE. Adverse effects of antimalarials. An update. Drug Safety. 1993;8:295-311.

81 Lange WR, Frankenfield DL, Moriarty-Sheehan M, Contoreggi CS, Frame JD. No evidence for chloroquine-associated retinopathy among missionaries on long-term malaria chemoprophylaxis. American Journal of Tropical Medicine & Hygiene. 1994;51:389-92.

82 Overbosch D. Post-marketing surveillance: adverse events during long-term use of atovaquone/proguanil for travelers to malaria-endemic countries. Journal of Travel Medicine. 2003;10(Suppl 1):S16-S20.